Advance Praise for RO(K BOTTOM AND FAITHLESS

"My first few months of a thirty-two-year career in law enforcement taught me never to be surprised at the horrific things people do to the ones they supposedly love. In fact, after several responses to calls of domestic violence, I became jaded, believing there were many more cases of domestic violence going unreported.

"So, with this jaundiced, suspicious perspective, how did I miss knowing that a dear friend, coworker, and high-performing law enforcement officer was herself a victim of domestic violence?

"Susan's daring, heart-wrenching story is one of strength, love, and bravery, with an appropriate ending to a horrific first marriage. With a reconstructed foundation built on faith, friends, and family, Susan shares her pain, the flawed reasoning that kept her in a damaging and demoralizing relationship, and how she found the strength to rise above it.

"But her book also quietly exposes how 'we'—the friends, family, and coworkers of abused and abusers—can be truly blind to what goes on behind closed doors.

"Susan's page-turning, hopeful exposé is a testament that even law enforcement officers, highly-educated executives, and other leaders are not immune to the lies of abusers, but gives hope of freedom to those who have been held in that harrowing grip."

—Colleen McGuire
  Brigadier General, US Army (Retired)
  Former Provost Marshal General of the Army; Commander,
  Criminal Investigations Command; Commandant, United
  States Disciplinary Barracks (Federal Penitentiary)

"Sue Parisher's book is a compelling account of one woman's journey of abuse—from victim to survivor. This is an easy-to-read introduction to domestic violence based on Sue's own story. Like the title suggests, it dispels myths and is faithful to the Christian Scriptures."

—Nancy Nason-Clark, PhD, FRSC
    Professor Emerita, University of New Brunswick
    Director, the RAVE Project, www.theraveproject.org

DEFEATING THE LIES OF
DOMESTIC ABUSE WITH
GOD'S TRUTH

ROCK BOTTOM AND FAITHLESS

SUE PARISHER WITH REBECCA DAVIS

Post Hill
PRESS

A SAVIO REPUBLIC BOOK
An Imprint of Post Hill Press
ISBN: 978-1-64293-191-4
ISBN (eBook): 978-1-64293-192-1

Author Photo by Chad Winstead

Scripture quotations taken from The Holy Bible, New International Version NIV. Copyright (c) 1973, 1978, 1984, 2011 by Biblica, Inc. Used by permission.

All people, locations, events, and situations are portrayed to the best of the author's memory. While all of the events described are true, many names and identifying details have been changed to protect the privacy of the people involved.

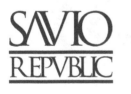 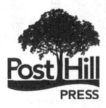

posthillpress.com
New York • Nashville
Published in the United States of America

To my mom
I am so sorry you passed away without knowing any of this.
I hated all those times I prioritized my emotional
and physical safety over being honest with you.
I know how much this secret strained our relationship.
I look forward to the day when we can laugh and smile together.
Love, Sue

TABLE OF CONTENTS

PART THREE
LIES LEADING UP TO THE NERVOUS BREAKDOWN

PART FOUR
FINAL LIES BLOCKING A LIFE OF PEACE

FOREWORD

Branson Sheets, lead pastor
  Covenant Church, Greenville, North Carolina

I'd seen Sue sitting out in the crowd in our church. She's probably like a lot of people in large congregations with multiple services: anonymous until they decide they don't want to be any longer.

One day she introduced herself to me. She seemed like a nice woman, you know, normal enough. Then she told me she was writing a book on her story of domestic violence. She asked if I knew of any ministry to such people at our church. She asked if I knew of any resources available in the community. Sue asked a lot of questions, and frankly, I was uncomfortable, and I had very few answers for her.

This conversation was the beginning of my understanding that Sue Parisher was recovering from years of cruel abuse. I remember thinking to myself, this woman doesn't look like someone who has been or even could have been abused. She was a lieutenant colonel in the U.S. Army. Could she really have been a victim of something like this?

The answer is yes.

This book tells Sue's courageous journey from an abuse victim who felt trapped in an unending cycle to a victorious woman who discovered the truth about God's love for her and her value as a person.

And let me tell you, *Rock Bottom and Faithless* is a great book. It walks through many painful episodes from earlier in her life when lies embedded in her thoughts from years of abuse were front and center in her thinking. She then shares how God began to reveal glimpses of truth as she began to see the lies for what they were. Every time I turned a page, I celebrated with Sue as she talked about a lie she used to believe about herself but now saw past to see herself the way her Heavenly Father sees her.

I am so proud of Sue. She is a courageous woman who has labored to overcome the effects of an abusive spouse. I also know that she has labored many years to be able to offer every word of this book as a tool to help other women see that they don't have to live in the pain and despair of abuse either.

What an incredible resource for those suffering from domestic violence! My prayer is that this book will give victims of abuse the courage to take steps away from their abusers.

It's also an incredible resource for everybody else. What Sue describes in this book might be going on in your family, your neighborhood, or your church family. Her story demonstrates that domestic abuse can be hard to spot, hard to admit, and hard for others to believe, and yet it goes on every day in numbers that are staggering.

I wonder how many more "Sues" there are out there in my congregation. Before reading this book, I probably wouldn't have noticed or even thought about that question. But now I understand domestic abuse in a way I never understood it before. Now when it appears in my congregation, I'm much better prepared to see, to listen, to believe, and to help those who have been harmed by its effects, to help them overcome the lies and walk in the truth of Jesus Christ.

Pastor Branson Sheets

INTRODUCTION

Tom gripped my neck in a choke hold, raising me high enough off the floor that my feet dangled freely.

"I don't know why I put up with such a moron," he hissed.

Just before I passed out from his grip around my neck, he released me, watching me flop to the ground, gasping for air.

"Stupid. Incompetent. Idiot."

Each epithet was punctuated with a kick to my stomach.

I curled up into a fetal position and covered my face.

"Stay out of my sight!" he roared. "You disgust me!"

He stomped out of the room.

As soon as I was sure he was gone, I crawled toward the door, sobbing. I reached up and locked it, and then went back down on my knees.

After twenty-one years of trying to manage my abusive husband, I knew I couldn't handle this situation any more. If he had killed me that night, I was sure he could have come up with an explanation that few people would have questioned. He was so convincing.

But I couldn't die. I had to stay alive for the sake of my children.

So as I knelt on that floor, tears streaming down my face, I desperately tried to reconnect with God.

God, I know I've been gone over twenty-one years, but I'm ready now to have you in my life. If you allow me to stay alive today, I promise I'll get myself and the kids away from him.

Every day for the next thirty days I prayed this same prayer. I didn't know what else to do. My secret double life had become unbearable.

———◆———

This incident marked the beginning of my *physical* escape from a twenty-one-year marriage full of emotional, physical, and sexual abuse.

Escaping the mental and emotional abuse has taken far longer.

Lies, lies, and more lies, embedded so deep in my mind that they became my own truths. I didn't know I had become so brainwashed that my abuser's thoughts controlled my actions, my beliefs, and my entire existence. I didn't know I had become a puppet, being manipulated by the embedded lies my abuser had convinced me were true.

Here I was, so confused about how my life had gotten so out of control, crying out to the God who I believed had allowed all of this pain to happen in my life.

I could no longer hide behind denial, hoping my marriage would return to the happier times of the past. It was there on my knees, sobbing hysterically, where I first began to try and relinquish control of the mess my world had become.

But before I could recover from the lies embedded within my brainwashed mind, I had to identify them. Then I could develop a plan to counter each lie, seeing truth more clearly, and appropriating God's help in defeating them.

I hope that the lessons I share—the lies and how I defeated them—from my eleven-year journey from domestic abuse victim to survivor will…

- ⊚ give you an idea of what to expect during this transition to domestic violence survivor;

- ⊚ help you break the stronghold of your abuser's embedded lies on your thoughts and actions;

- help lessen the aggravating impact your abuser has on your world;

- help break the secrecy of recovery, so those in your world will be better able to understand and assist;

- strengthen your relationship with God, therefore allowing His grace to provide you with strength and peace.

Becoming a domestic violence survivor has for me meant being free and open to living again. It means I can make decisions, build trusting relationships, and even feel love. It means the thoughts in my head are mine and mine alone.

With the emotional abuse removed from my mind, God's grace and love have taken over with a calmness and peace I never before thought possible.

I pray that my story of overcoming the lies implanted by domestic abuse will help you on your own path in defeating deceptions and reclaiming your future and hope. If so, then I thank God for what He has taught me, even in the midst of pain.

Blessings,
Sue

PART ONE

LIES FROM WITHIN THE ABUSE

CHAPTER 1

VALENTINE'S DAY

My first Valentine's Day with Tom was in 1987, back when we were dating. It was a memory I held in secret and pulled out every once in a while to try to soothe my fears and pain.

We were stationed in Korea at the time, and he couldn't decide what to get me. So he got me one of everything.

Perfume…

a big box of candy…

flowers…

jewelry…

a huge, beautiful card…

and a six-foot-tall stuffed polar bear.

I was overwhelmed. I had never felt so loved. Imagine being showered with so many gifts so early in a relationship—this was surely a sign of greater showers of affection to come!

He loved me so much. I felt so lucky.

I held that memory during the moments I watched his steady breathing after he had fallen asleep…minutes after screaming filthy names at me.

On our third Valentine's Day, when we were snowed in at Fort Lewis, Washington, Tom walked to the store a mile and a half in the snow, telling me it was to get me flowers and a gift. (I later found out the real purpose of the walk was to get himself cigarettes, but I learned to easily forget that part of the memory.)

How thoughtful of him. We were now married, and he was still showering me with affection.

These were the memories I held onto when I hunched in a corner trying to get control over my terrified breathing after he had stomped out of the room after kicking me.

He bought me a beautiful dress once, and I felt so pretty in it, so different from the rigor of my army uniform.

He fixed me a romantic dinner once when I was pregnant with our first child. I can still close my eyes and remember it, red roses in the vase, romantic music instead of the ESPN that was usually blaring. As I would later realize this was the only time he acknowledged how special it was that I was carrying his child. I cherished the memory of this night.

Three or four times he bought me a bouquet of "I'm sorry" flowers. They always brightened my mood as I proudly displayed them in the kitchen (even though something in the back of my mind said they were sending the message that I was supposed to ignore all his bad behavior).

For the longest time I thought the flowers meant he regretted his actions and that he was going to try harder to not repeat the same insensitive things.

I held onto these memories like small jewels in the back of a chaotic junk drawer.

"There are never enough clean clothes around here. Why can't you keep this house in order? You didn't use enough starch ironing my uniform! What kind of garbage do you want me to eat, you idiot?"

I knew other army husbands of army wives ironed their own uniforms. I wouldn't have minded ironing if he had helped with the house, or the kitchen, or the shopping, or—later in the marriage—the kids…. But he relaxed on the couch watching sports while he ordered me to iron and do all the other housework and take care of the children too. And if I completed my list, I was instructed to sit on the couch with him, watching endless hours of sports that I was definitely not interested in.

But still, my mind would flit back to those few thoughtful memories, those precious jewels from the past.

Maybe one day, if I was good enough, that nice guy would come back.

THE LIE: IF I TRY HARD ENOUGH, THE NICE GUY WILL RETURN

Sadly, those examples were the only "nice guy" stories I can remember from our twenty-one-years of marriage.

By the time our second child arrived, Tom was so tired of buying "I'm sorry" flowers that the last batch of flowers he gave me came with a huge disclaimer.

Tom was not going to apologize anymore.

At the time I thought for sure this was another one of his rambling, spontaneous statements. I never believed he meant he was never going to buy me flowers again. There was no way he really meant that.

But he did. He told me he wasn't wasting money on flowers anymore, and he meant it. Apparently, I didn't deserve them.

But I continued in denial. My husband wasn't so bad. After all, he was an army officer. People throughout the military units we were assigned to respected him so much. Those horrible stories in the news about men abusing their wives were terrible, but thank goodness my marriage was fixable. My husband was really a good guy—that's what everyone in our military units told me.

And after all, Tom used make me laugh. He used to make me feel special. He used to convince me that I was the most important person in his life.

Even as I saw what was happening in our marriage, I didn't have words for it. For so long I denied the truth and suppressed the feelings of how horribly wrong things were. I became so busy reacting, fixing, anticipating, and responding to Tom's moods that I never took (or had) the time to stop and realize what was going on. Any free minutes in my thoughts were devoted to trying to anticipate what might happen next or trying to respond to the new crisis that had arisen.

It must be my fault, and I'll keep trying harder. Someday my world will become better. Surely any day now, this pain and terror will be a thing of the past.

Happier days will surely be coming soon.

At least that's what my denial convinced me of.

A GLIMMER OF TRUTH

It would be years later until I understood how powerful my denial was at pulling me through my years of pain and suffering.

A pivotal point in the beginning of my journey out of denial was finally realizing that my world was not going to change. At various moments, this truth shone on me with great clarity.

As the years passed and I kept trying harder while the abuse kept getting worse, I began to realize that the great guy I married wasn't returning.

The time he almost killed me was the clincher.

As the memory of Tom's attempt to kill me continuously replayed in my mind, I started to realize that whether I wanted to or not, I must now make drastic changes in my life. I had to start accepting the reality that I could no longer remain in my current situation or my children would end up motherless. The changes had to start now.

When my mother and sister found out I was divorcing Tom, they were glad for me to get away from that monstrous man and hoped that the "old me" would return.

But they really had no idea of the magnitude of the evil I was escaping. Denial played a part even in that silence. It would be years before I understood this lie I clutched so tightly.

SEEING TRUTH CLEARLY

As the years have passed and I've received counseling for multiple issues, including denial, I've become able to see some important truths about being a domestic violence victim. Denial:

- kept me loyal to my abuser;

- impeded my decision-making abilities;

- compartmentalized the bad times, making the return of the "nice" guy seem possible;

- held onto the false belief that true love and companionship would return and triumph;

- kept me from feeling confident that I could ever take care of myself and my children;

- confused the formation of exit strategies and safety plans;

- produced a strange and toxic mix of overwhelming anxiety, fear, and second-guessing.

Although the world of denial that I lived in with Tom was a crazy, anxiety-ridden world, it was *my* world that I had been conditioned to. Even if it felt unsafe, it felt *familiar*.

Moving into the world of the unknown was extremely frightening. But it was worth it. Over and over again I reminded myself that almost anything was better than the horrible existence of being married to Tom.

CHAPTER 2

THANKSGIVING DINNER

Everyone else seemed to be having fun at Grandma's house on Thanksgiving. Laughter, clatter in the kitchen, guys sneaking pieces of turkey while Grandpa was carving the bird and Grandma lovingly surveyed her grandchildren scurrying all around.

Three generations of family together created a feeling of love and acceptance. Everyone seemed relaxed, hungry, and content.

As the buffet line opened on the kitchen counter, family members squeezed in to get first helpings of their favorite dishes.

My first time through the line, I prepared my two-year-old's plate. I navigated through the crowd, worked my way over to the drink table, and then to where he sat. I leaned over and cut up his food.

My second time through the buffet line, I fixed my four-year-old's plate. The crowd had died down a little, so navigating back to the kids' table was easier. After I cut up his food, I noticed everyone was already enjoying the amazing feast.

Leaning into the living room, I asked Tom, "What do you want to eat?" After attentively listening to his requests I turned back to what was now an empty kitchen.

"Why aren't you getting your own food for yourself?" Tom's sister asked him. "Sue is obviously busy with your two little boys."

Tom proudly replied, "Oh, my wife loves to make my plate, don't you, honey?"

Of course, dear.

By the time I made my own plate of food, the crowd was gathering for seconds. Embarrassed and angry, I was reminded once again of how out of control my waiting on my husband had become.

THE LIE: I AM MY HUSBAND'S SLAVE

But this bizarre servanthood, so public at Thanksgiving dinner, was a regular occurrence at home.

Tom would sit on the couch watching ESPN and suddenly yell, "Where's my supper? I said I want it now!"

But I was trying to remember, *did he want teriyaki sauce with his onions, or was it something else? Which drink was he going to want tonight? Do I have the right serving sizes on the dinner plate? Oh dear, the onions are touching the rice. I don't want him throwing this perfectly prepared meal across the room. I definitely don't have time to clean up another mess tonight.*

But I could never, ever do it right.

A GLIMMER OF TRUTH

After I was able to get out, trying to keep myself and my children safe, there were so many lies I had to untangle. "I am his slave" was a foundational one from which many others sprang.

In those early days after getting out, when I wanted to reminisce about the few good times I had with Tom, I had to learn to counter any positive memories before they could settle in. As quickly as possible I needed to remember Tom as the mean and cruel slave master he actually was. Even though it was painful and difficult to do this at first, it was essential for my safety and the safety of my children that I remembered the life of slavery he had forced on me.

CHAPTER 3

FILES ON THE FLOOR

Tom's large frame filled the doorway as he jerked open the drawers of the filing cabinet.

"Couldn't answer such a simple question." His mutter rose in volume. "What makes you think any of this tax information is right? Any of it at all? What a fuckin moron."

He sneered in disdain at the file folders I had painstakingly sorted and neatly laid out on the floor. Salary information. Mortgage information. Uniform expenses. Charity deductions.

Still kneeling amidst them, I glanced down in despair. Only moments ago I had been so proud of what I had accomplished. I flinched as he continued.

"I'll bet this whole tax return is wrong, you stupid idiot."

I made myself as small as possible on the floor as I watched him, standing there in the doorway at the filing cabinet. Almost in slow motion, it seemed, I saw him pull out each of the remaining file folders from the drawer and toss each one up in the air. He didn't bother to watch the papers scatter and float all over the room the way I did. He was busy pulling out the next one, and the next, and the next.

I watched, in a daze, holding back the tears.

Again and again. Through each one of the three filing cabinet drawers, until the room was so covered with paper I couldn't even see the floor.

"That's what you get for doing it wrong, bitch," he roared. "Next time you'll do it right. And don't come out of this room until you put this all back together. Correctly!"

He strode away, back up the stairs.

Quickly, quickly, I thought. *I need to clean this up. My two little boys are hungry and I need to fix supper.*

THE LIE: I AM INCOMPETENT

My life was so confusing. Most people would say I was successful during my twenty-one years on active duty in the army; after all, I retired a lieutenant colonel.

My leaders and subordinates thought I was competent; my annual evaluations and promotions confirmed that I did a commendable job.

But truth be told, I never felt like I was doing a good job, nor did I believe I earned the various accolades or promotions I received. My internal conflict assured me I was a complete imbecile and somehow everyone just hadn't seen it yet. I felt like everybody else knew what they were doing and I was the only idiot bouncing around what other people did or said. I always believed it was the great officers and soldiers I worked with who made me appear successful.

This lie of being incompetent was drilled into me over and over, day after day, year after year, for all twenty-one years that Tom and I were together.

"You are so stupid."

"You're so ignorant you don't know something as simple as *that?*"

It didn't matter what it was. Tom's comments toward me always showcased my obvious ignorance and stupidity.

This was Tom's drill: Relentlessly, ceaselessly, drilling into me that I was an incompetent moron. Continually challenging me to improve "for my own good." Treating me like a small child who hadn't learned her lesson yet, and might never learn it because she was just. So. Stupid. When I was at home, I might as well have been wearing a dunce cap.

Imagine the confusion and awkwardness I felt while being the warden at the Department of Defense prison in Germany. Prison warden by day; prisoner in my home at night.

For so many years my life felt split. High-achieving supervisor at work; imbecilic, moronic captive at home.

The "home me" felt like it must be the real me and the "work me" felt like an act, a put-on.

A GLIMMER OF TRUTH

It was years before I finally realized that Tom wasn't interested in helping me improve or learn; he just wanted to hurt me and would find any excuse to do so.

The light dawned one day when he was "instructing" me from the living room couch on how to make him lunch.

"Hey, make me a peanut butter and jelly sandwich," he yelled. "I'm starving."

I immediately stopped what I was doing and carefully prepared a peanut butter and jelly sandwich and took it to him.

"You *know* I hate grape jelly! I only eat strawberry jelly, you stupid fool. And where the hell is my dessert?"

I immediately fixed a new sandwich and brought it to Tom along with a Twinkie.

"In what world does a peanut butter and jelly sandwich go with a Twinkie?" he hollered. "Twinkies are for kids. And since when do I like my sandwich cut corner to corner? You idiot, make me a new sandwich and cut it top to bottom and bring me another dessert, not something stupid that the kids eat."

That day something clicked inside of me.

I finally realized this was not about my being incompetent. Each time I had done what he had said. But he had purposely withheld information from me so I'd be sure to get it wrong. *It was about him wanting to keep me anxious and off balance.*

That afternoon was when the light began to dawn. I realized it didn't matter how many times I made this sandwich or picked out a dessert, nothing I brought him was going to please him. *The only thing that pleased him was that he was destroying my belief that I could do anything right.*

My abuser wasn't interested in "helping me become a better wife"; he just intended to control my responses to his demands. He wasn't interested in what I was doing at all; all he was interested in was ensuring I knew that he was in charge and ungrateful for anything I did for him.

SEEING TRUTH CLEARLY

It was when I was able to give words to the truth that I was finally able to bring both parts of my life together.

I was not incompetent.

Instead, Tom was a cruel man who wanted to hurt me, and he wanted to make up excuses to do it.

I was manipulated, controlled, abused, and afraid.

But I was not incompetent. My "work self" was, in fact, my real self.

Once I was able to get out from the abuse and the effects of the abuse (a very long journey!), I could see that.

In fact, I could finally begin to see, here and there, more and more evidence that I was indeed a capable person. As I have continued through the years of recovery and have successfully navigated challenging life situations, I've seen it.

Incompetent people don't survive the level of abuse I did.

I am not incompetent.

I am capable.

SPEAKING TRUTH:
THE POWER OF A NAME

During my recovery from domestic violence, it has seemed that my patterns of thinking have been the last things to change. It took me far too long, but I finally came to a place where I was able to realize that one of the most powerful ways to establish control of my thoughts was through *names*.

THE LEVEL OF RESPECT CONVEYED BY A NAME

Titles are used throughout our world to establish legitimate power, responsibilities, and boundaries for individuals. When we see a person's title (president, CEO, doctor, executive, or assistant) we can develop an idea of what that person's responsibilities are. The title can also indicate a level of authority. It often generates automatic respect, respect that isn't necessarily deserved.

THE POWER OF THE NAMES I WAS CALLED

It seemed that in my world, the exact opposite was true. The derogatory names my abuser conveyed on me signified my lack of worth, lack of value, and lack of importance to him.

Without my even realizing it, the negative names I was called slowly took away my self-esteem, self-worth, and trust in my ability to be a wife, mother, daughter, and coworker.

While the names my abuser called me stripped me of my capacity to be myself, they simultaneously provided him with power and control over me.

THE POWER OF THE NAMES I CHOOSE TO USE

I now understand that what I name a person indicates the level of respect that I have for him or her. But I actually didn't realize the power in a name until one day when my sister was reading some of my writings. She wanted to know why I was referring to Tom as my ex-husband.

"He's your abuser," she said.

And she was correct; Tom should always be referred to as my abuser.

But, without someone coaching me toward this deliberate mental switch, I struggled aimlessly for control of my emotions toward my abuser.

I needed to properly identify the abuse for what it was: I was a domestic violence victim and Tom was my abuser.

Now that I look back, I am amazed at how powerful a name can be. Even without speaking the name, recognizing that I can choose what name I can use provided me a new degree of emotional control.

When I began calling Tom "my abuser" instead of "my ex-husband," it quickly reminded me of the horrible situation I was trying to escape.

I eventually realized that the name I used for my abuser identified where I was in my journey to recovery. Here are the names I have called my abuser during my years of recovery.

Tom: This is the person I fell in love with and committed my life to.

Ex-husband: This is a neutral term. I'm not a bad person just because I'm an ex-wife.

Abuser: This is a better representation of who Tom was to me, but this has to come with the acknowledgment that he hurt me. This word was hard for me to start using because I had to admit that I wasn't going to be able to make him happy.

MY DAWNING UNDERSTANDING

John 8:44 tells us that Satan is the father of lies.[1] As I *speak* truth and *believe* truth and by the power of the Holy Spirit *rest in* the truth, I am waging warfare against him.

As I have chosen names that accurately reflect who Tom chose to be and the path that Tom chose to follow, I am *speaking* truth. As I have allowed these truths to sink into my soul, even though they have caused grief, I am *believing* truth.

As I receive the names that Jesus wants to call me, such as His beloved, His sheep, and His daughter, I am *resting in* truth.

I can combat the lies that were thrust into my soul by that follower of the devil, my abuser. And one of the ways I do that is by knowing and using the appropriate names, because there is so much power in the names we choose to use.

---

1   Jesus said to the Pharisees, "You are of your father the devil, and your will is to do your father's desires. He was a murderer from the beginning, and does not stand in the truth, because there is no truth in him. When he lies, he speaks out of his own character, for he is a liar and the father of lies."

CHAPTER 4

WoMAN'S WoRK

"You're an idiot if you think I'm going to help with those," Tom sneered at our newborn baby's diaper. He turned his back to me and focused on the sports on TV. It didn't matter that my work day had been longer than his.

Our new little one cried out in the night…again. Tom rolled over, snoring loudly. I got the message and crawled out of bed…again. It didn't matter that I had to be up at 5:30 in the morning to get ready for work the next day.

I was the one who did all the childcare, all the food shopping, all the cooking and cleaning, all the laundry, all the school obligations for our children, and all their doctor appointments. And all this in spite of working full-time.

In fact, everything about raising our children was up to me—except showing them off to others. When our first child was a few months old Tom carried him around like a prized possession, proudly showing him off to everyone at our military unit's soccer game.

But as soon as we were in the car, he started complaining about how the dirty diaper smelled, saying I'd better hustle to get that stink out of the car.

Every work day was like this.

Eventually, they rolled into one big mess of constant tension, stress, and yelling. Eventually, I became overwhelmingly tired.

And mad.

And jealous.

Unfortunately, my feelings started to show in my clanging and banging things around. Now I was being yelled at for being "bitchy" on top of all the other names he was calling me.

The black hole I lived in continued to grow deeper.

THE LIE: EVERYTHING IS MY RESPONSIBILITY

My abuser not only pushed all responsibility of our world onto me, but also blamed me for everything that went wrong in his life.

And over the years I accepted the blame, wearing it like a fifty-pound weight strapped to my back, convinced that it was my responsibility to carry it.

This undeserved blame weighed me down so strongly that my ability to see what was really going on disappeared.

And, since I was to blame for Tom's poor decision-making, it only made sense that I was also responsible for the consequences.

This led me to believe that the faster I fixed the fallout of a poor decision, the less chance I would have of being yelled at and blamed for the situation. Time was always of the essence. It was vitally important that a situation get cleaned up before the next negative event occurred.

Yet I also know what a mess Tom's poor decisions and bad choices created. Sometimes they created an expensive situation that we couldn't afford. Sometimes they created tension between us (like when I was promoted to lieutenant colonel and he wasn't).

Or, the worst, when Tom's wallowing in the aftermath of a poor decision impacted his relationship with the children. A bad week at work followed by a night out drinking almost always guaranteed he would cancel whatever plans our children had with him on Saturday. Our two little boys never understood.

Yet I took to heart all the blame Tom imposed on me for his horrible week. My self-imposed guilt caused me to cover up the boys' disappointment on another Saturday morning event their dad canceled.

Cleaning up Tom's messes became another item on my long list of things to do each week.

A GLIMMER OF TRUTH

It was with my second long-term therapist, seven years after I was separated from Tom, that I began to understand that it's not my responsibility to make everything perfect for those around me.

It took me a long time to accept the fact that when other people make poor decisions that impact their lives, I'm not to blame for the fallout.

My abuser is responsible for his poor decisions and unwise choices.

What a powerful, impactful statement! My abuser was responsible for what he did or didn't do. His poor decision-making skills were not my fault, and I didn't—and I do not—have to bear that responsibility.

I am responsible for my decisions and choices. I am responsible for what I do. I am not responsible for him.

CHAPTER 5

ABANDONED IN THE HOSPITAL

"God, help my daughter!"

I was sitting in the Intensive Care Unit with my sleeping three-year-old, who had just received a bone marrow transplant for leukemia.

"God, please help my little girl!"

Night after night, week after week, watching the weary hours pass.

Here I was, living in the secret world of domestic violence, and I found that my baby girl had been diagnosed with leukemia. Though at first the chemotherapy seemed to be working, after a year of continuous treatments, my little girl's cancer had returned, vigorously. Leukemia cells were spreading throughout her three-year-old body.

I reached out and gripped her little hand, gazing at her tiny bald head on the hospital pillow, marveling at how her thin body lay dwarfed in the huge hospital bed, watching the steady rise and fall of her chest.

How much more could one person possibly be expected to take? Daily I was verbally or physically assaulted by my husband, and now one of our children was battling cancer?

I couldn't think straight. There I was, trying to learn everything I could about childhood cancer, while becoming a primary caregiver, raising two boys under the age of eight, and being a battered wife.

At times, I literally could not breathe.

"Are you there, God? Will you help her?"

I shifted uncomfortably in the chair and looked around the room at the technical equipment and silently flashing lights, focusing on the now-familiar hospital noises.

This was a safe place, at least physically. He wouldn't hit me here. Besides, his visits were rare.

His visits were also obnoxious and hungover, disgusting and volatile. And random, unexpected.

But infrequent, at least.

No one else came at all.

What a lonely place.

"Is there an angel that will help her?" I prayed. "A Leukemia angel?"

Someone.

I used to know God long ago, I thought. *Oh, it was so long ago, so, so long ago.* I rubbed my forehead.

"You can help her, God. You can protect her," I prayed out loud. "Please help her, Leukemia angels."

For two weeks, I prayed this way in that lonely hospital room.

Then, one afternoon, out of nowhere, a thought came to me.

I'm going to tell my daughter's doctor about the way my husband is treating me. I'm going to tell him!

Her doctor would be here at dinnertime. He always was, every time he was on call. I could set my watch by it.

Telling my daughter's oncology doctor would be dangerous, I knew, but I would finally get some help. He would know what to do. I'd tell him everything and even show him the bruises on my arm to prove it.

I was going to take the first step to putting an end to the madness that had become my world.

So that afternoon, I sat back, closed my eyes, and waited.

Today would be the beginning of something different.

But he didn't stop by my daughter's room during evening hours!

7:30 p.m. passed. 8:00 p.m. 9:00 p.m. 10:00 p.m.

On the very night I decided to ask for help, the one person I trusted to ask for that help didn't show up.

Why would this happen? On the very day I was ready to tell my terrible secret?

Then the thought flashed into my mind. It must have been God. God must have done this to me. He was the one, I thought, who had led me to build up hope, only to let me down.

I was ready to tell about my abuse, but God prevented it. Somehow this seemed intentional and cruel.

Did God want my abuser to win? Did that mean He wanted cancer to win?

Then I became overwhelmingly afraid. Was my abuse so dangerous that no one could be trusted with my secret?

I was heartbroken and defeated. And the Lie seeped back up.

My punishments for old sins were not over.

THE LIE: I DESERVE TO BE PUNISHED

This Lie was so far back in my mind, buried so deep in the foundation of my thinking, that it had become a bedrock belief. When I sat there in the hospital, I couldn't even put words to it.

It was years before I could vocalize this Lie.

"I deserve to be punished" was never a spoken thought. It was just inherent knowledge, like, "I am a human being." Not the kind of thing you think about it, because it's just so self-evident.

This cruel-seeming set of circumstances in the hospital confirmed this "truth" that was already integrated into my entire being.

I *knew* I deserved the bruises, the yelling, the constant correction, being treated like a child. Every time. With every punishment or bad experience. Day after day, week after week, year after year. With every bad thing that happened, this was my mantra.

As a teenager I had sinned terribly, and the guilt I carried cried out for punishment. I *needed* to be punished. Being abandoned in the hospital while I harbored this terrible secret of abuse—it must be one more punishment.

I knew. So at some level it all made sense.

It made sense, too, the time when Tom was driving and I was giving directions, the time I told him to go left when I should have said right. It made sense that he would throw a milkshake at me for such a stupid mistake. When the milkshake flew everywhere, it made sense that he would tell me my punishment was that I couldn't leave the car until it was all cleaned up.

I rolled with the punches, literally, and did what I needed to do.

I deserved it.

When the abuse increased threefold after our daughter's cancer diagnosis, from awful to horrific, I hated it and feared it. But still.

I deserved it.

Through all the countless bruises, the rages, the fear, the endless punishments.

I deserved it.

When Tom and I were finally separated that didn't mean this mindset instantly changed. Well-meaning friends and family told me to just ignore him (or in today's terms, to block him). To them it seemed so easy, so straightforward.

They didn't understand that I had been so brainwashed that I knew if I ignored him there would be another punishment.

And of course, I would deserve it.

A GLIMMER OF LIGHT AND HOPE

It wasn't until years later, after I was free from the abuse and hesitantly groping for God again, that a chink began to form in the armor of "I deserve it."

A couple of years after my divorce from Tom, I met my current husband, Randy, who is a man driven by faith in God instead of selfishness. During our dating years as I grew to love him, I also learned to trust him with my deepest secrets.

I remember one Sunday morning Randy and I heard the pastor preach something that stirred my heart.

Since Jesus Christ has borne the punishment for our sins, through faith in Him we are forgiven of our sins.

After church on that beautiful sunny spring day, Randy and I drove to his parents' house for brunch, but during the entire forty-five-minute drive, I simply gazed out the window.

Something deep inside my heart was conflicted and struggling.

God says that when we trust Jesus for our salvation, we are forgiven for our sins, but there was no way He meant I was forgiven for the horrible things I had done.

The pain within my heart overwhelmed me. I knew God had to be using a sin meter. The only people He forgave were the ones who committed the lesser sins.

I had to find out the truth. When we arrived at the house, we just sat in the car silently for a few moments. Finally, I was able to quietly share my confusion and why I was sure God was punishing me through my daughter's illness.

After listening to my pain and struggle, Randy wrapped his arms around me. It felt as though God was personally telling me the truth for the first time.

Now I've learned that God will correct me, teach me, and even rebuke me, but He does not punish me. Jesus has taken all that for me.

SEEING TRUTH CLEARLY

After years of therapy and faith building, I am able to believe this powerful truth: through faith in Jesus Christ, God has forgiven me of my sins, so I can forgive myself too. I now realize that in God's world, life doesn't work in a karmic fashion, with evil always being punished in this life. Sometimes, people who have chosen evil get away with their wickedness.

And sometimes people who love God suffer.

Suffering under abuse, or suffering from my daughter's cancer, none of it was about a "deserving" punishment.

God doesn't work that way.

No, He doesn't always stop evil. Yes, many difficult circumstances have come into my life. (But He did answer my prayer to deliver my daughter from leukemia, and more than fourteen years later she is strong and healthy!)

One thing I have learned in my faith path is that Jesus has died for me, and when I trusted in Him for my salvation, He made me free. He has freed me from sin and freed me from the punishment for sin.

Yes, God has allowed many difficult experiences in my life, but in every experience He has wanted to help me and draw me to Himself, with love and patience.

As I have continued to grow in my faith and receive good counseling, I have been able to see it more and more clearly.

I could let go of "I deserve it."

CHAPTER 6

PRISONER AT HOME

I stood in the bedroom doorway, dressed in my uniform, ready to leave for my job as warden at the army prison. I glanced back at Tom, still gently snoring.

Just last week during a parole board hearing, I became aware of a prisoner's crime. The man had received a dishonorable discharge with loss of pay and benefits and was currently being held in the facility.

And just last night Tom had done a very similar thing to me.

Sodomy. That's what Tom was doing to me. He didn't care that I hated it and feared it and that it hurt me physically. He didn't care.

Why is it okay for a man to do things to his wife against her will, when outside of marriage he would be arrested for it? It didn't make sense. It shouldn't be happening.

But as I pulled the car out of the driveway and headed to the prison, I thought about how my alternative to enduring these despicable acts of violence didn't seem much more appealing.

First, I would have to actually tell my story while trying to stay safe. It made me shudder with fear and shame just to think of it.

And then if I was believed and Tom was disciplined the way the man in the prison was, all his income and benefits would be lost.

Was it worth it to go through the pain of that disruption to my world? My boys were four and two years old. I still had years left on active duty. How could I possible stay safe and still care for them? Who could I possibly trust with my growing secret?

As I flashed my warden badge on the way into the prison, I pondered my situation. Surely I was everything Tom said I was: incompetent, useless, stupid, weak, and worse. How could I ever believe I was capable of being a single parent while upholding my obligations on active duty?

There was no way out.

I decided on what I thought was my best course of action: Try harder to make my abuser happy. Control the kids so they wouldn't bother him. Shut my mouth and tiptoe around him so as not to cause arguments. Pick up the house more. Get the laundry done and put away faster. Cook his favorite foods more often. Never interrupt him when he's watching sports on TV. And let him keep doing the awful deeds to me in the bedroom.

When my daughter was diagnosed with leukemia, I felt like the imprisonment became secured even further. Since my abuser was the primary insurance provider, not only would he always know where my daughter's doctors were, but he also controlled the availability of treatment.

And as the final straw, I was sure I wouldn't be accepted at a domestic violence shelter with my daughter so sick.

I knew I was trapped; there was no way I could get free.

THE LIE: I'M TRAPPED

All the other lies of my marriage that had weighed down on me through the years, all of them came together in the one enslaving lie of "I'm trapped."

- *"If I keep trying hard, the nice guy will return."* Well, I had tried and tried and tried, and he hadn't come back, so I must just be too stupid to do it right. After all, he told me that all the time.

- *"I am incompetent."* That seemed self-evident.

- *"I am my husband's slave."* I'll keep trying harder and doing better.

- *"Everything is my responsibility."* If I didn't do it, it wouldn't get done. So I had to be there.

- *"I deserve to be punished."* I wasn't worth any better life than what I was getting. Who was I to think I could possibly make a better life for myself and my children?

For so many years, my lack of self-confidence overpowered my ability to even remotely believe that there was a way I could safely leave my abuser and live a life without him. I believed I wasn't:

- able to survive on my own without his income,

- strong enough to fight the court battle and win custody of my children,

- able to convince a judge of what my abuser did to me,

- able to keep myself and my children safe during the separation,

- able to take care of my world without my abuser telling me what to do and when.

All these lies worked together to clamp shackles on my feet. There was no way I could escape.

A GLIMMER OF TRUTH

After my failed determination to tell my daughter's cancer doctor about the abuse, I stayed for three more years before my abuser's attempt to kill me (described in the introduction). Those three years are a blur of bruises, yelling, punishments, pain, and anxiety. As the children grew older and witnessed more, juggling the secret of the abuse became harder and harder.

But the day my abuser almost killed me was the day I knew I had to find the strength to get out of this trap. Obviously, my earlier ways of trying to manage the situation weren't working at all. After years of being abused, it was time for me to do something.

That night I crawled over to my bed, and like a little child, I kneeled with my hands neatly folded. I remember begging God for his assistance, promising that if He kept me alive tonight, I would do everything in my power to remove myself and my children from this horrible situation. I couldn't die without trying to free myself from my abuser's grip.

In the days, weeks, and months that followed that night, I planned my strategy for moving myself and my children away from my abuser.

Could I take care of my children and myself on my paycheck? Of course I could, and I did.

SEEING TRUTH CLEARLY

It was being brought to the brink of death that finally made me realize there was no good reason to stay in this trap.

First of all, my abuser not only did not love me—he actually despised me enough to kill me.

And, if I didn't break the cycle of domestic violence, I realized my two boys could become abusers themselves. After all, they had been witnessing my abuser's cruelty for years. (Later I read that men who witnessed their parents' domestic violence as children were twice as likely to abuse their wives compared with sons of nonviolent parents.)

Equally important, if my daughter continued to witness this type of abusive behavior, she could be in danger of learning to approve of it, to accept it, from men in her life.

I longed to keep my sons from doing to anyone else what was being done to me.

With God as my help, I was leaving my trap. I was escaping. The decision was monumental.

Though I had no idea the spiritual warfare that would continue to rage in my mind and heart, all I could see was that the door of denial was about to be opened, and my journey to recovering from domestic violence had begun.

PART TWO

LIES FROM THE EARLY DAYS OF GETTING OUT

CHAPTER 7

GUT PUNCH IN A SUB SHOP

Two years after my daughter's bone marrow transplant, while she was still under doctor's care and taking prescription medicine multiple times a day, my abuser took a job seven hours away. For an entire year he came home maybe four times.

I remember one of his rare trips home, he asked me to meet him at a local sub shop before he saw the children.

During that whole anxious year of being a single mom, this one encounter with Tom remains vivid, as if it happened yesterday. I remember his gray T-shirt, black shorts, and old flip-flops. I remember his unshaven face and the smell of cigarette smoke.

Mostly I remember his emotionless voice speaking words that slapped me in the face and punched me in the gut.

"We aren't going to make it together any more. I just wanted to let you know we need to get a divorce."

At that moment my world stopped cold in its tracks. I barely breathed. My ability to think vanished while anxiety and uncertainty immediately overwhelmed me. It took all I had to not throw up. My world was shattering.

I leaned in toward Tom and fought back the tears. "Please don't make this decision so fast," I pleaded. "Please reconsider. Don't leave the kids and me. Listen, if you'll just leave this job and move back home, I'll do anything you want. Anything."

I was 100 percent convinced that I was unable to think, act, or accomplish anything on my own. As I sat there in the sub shop with customers barely glancing our way, my mind flooded with the litany of my incompetencies that proved I couldn't survive without him.

He didn't know that every day, as I struggled to survive in his absence, I encountered new and confusing situations. The more unfamiliar situations arose, the more I doubted my ability to figure out what to do. I had grown so accustomed to Tom telling me what to do, how to do it, and when to do it, that I could not figure out how to do something on my own. I was raising three children under the age of twelve as a single parent, and I felt totally clueless.

How was I possibly going to survive without Tom telling me when to pay bills? How to enforce homework and chores? How to keep from making a mistake in the protocol for our daughter's recovery? Who was going to tell me when to take the two boys in for haircuts? Who was going to tell me how often the yard should be mowed? (I surely didn't want to ruin it like he told me I did at our house in Washington State.)

I would love to say that after this painful conversation I immediately figured out how to do all these things on my own. Unfortunately, at that time the strength of his emotional battering was still too overpowering for me.

Eventually, Tom did return from this job and move back home. I welcomed him back into our world with loving arms and a determination to do everything I could this time to make him want to stay, until the night he attempted to kill me.

THE LIE: SEPARATING MEANS MY WORLD WILL FALL APART

The sad fact is that my low self-esteem, second-guessing, confusion, and anxiety meant I was sure I couldn't function on my own.

I was frightened. I couldn't imagine a life without pain, suffering, and mental anguish. I couldn't imagine getting better physically, emotionally, or financially.

I couldn't think straight. My memory and decision-making abilities were reduced as Tom continuously told me how stupid, ignorant, and selfish I was. Surely, I really was all those things—my consistent mistakes and ridiculous incompetencies confirmed it.

When Tom and I finally did separate for good (after he attempted to kill me), I was overwhelmingly lonely and scared, concerned for my safety and that of my children. I was overwhelmed trying to make decisions on my own, trying to function without my abuser telling me what and how to do everything, without any financial support, all the while constantly looking over my shoulder for his impending arrival.

Most of all, I was overwhelmed with an inability to function. This came as a natural result of...

my shattered fairy-tale love story,

my financial stability ruined,

my becoming a single mom and not being able to raise my children in a traditional family environment.,

my abuser moving on with dating (was I jealous?) and enjoying his life,

my inability to concentrate at work,

my diminished ability to trust again.

Even one of these experiences would have caused me problems trying to cope in life. Combined, they destroyed any ability I had to function. Combined, they left me powerless and incapable of doing anything.

Even though my fear of dying kept me from sharing any of my horrors, I couldn't possibly express how I was feeling anyway. I would rather have just agreed with whatever someone told me to do than try to explore, understand, or express what I was feeling, much less get control of my thoughts.

Unable to open up about my past and current confusion, I continued to hide behind my misery without the support or understanding of my family or few acquaintances. Holding in all this confusion and pain, not sharing it with anyone, significantly increased my emotional confusion. I was still a "domestic violence victim" hiding in secrecy without even understanding what kind of mess I was stuck in.

Finally, for the first time in over twenty years, my ability to function came to a screeching halt.

A GLIMMER OF TRUTH

I am not an expert, but to me, this now sounds like depression, and I believe I needed professional help. I needed someone I could speak with comfortably. I needed to be honest about everything I was going through: the confusion, fears, darkness, guilt, and everything else. It was one of my biggest mistakes that I wasn't open about these things to professional counselors early on in my recovery.

People in my small world offered great tips for easing my depression. They told me I should eat better, walk more, and be grateful that I was separated from that horrible person who changed me into someone they didn't know anymore. Yes, I agree, too much processed sugar and not enough exercise was bad for me at the time, but I also believe these outsiders had no idea what I was going through and couldn't realize the magnitude of the confusion in my head.

One philosophy that did work for me was to "tackle the elephant one toe at a time." During those early recovery years, many competing life issues fought to overwhelm me: my finances, living situation, childcare, job, car maintenance, parents' health, divorce proceedings, and my children's health. When I tried to work on many projects at the same time, I felt like I was just running around in circles without really getting much of anything accomplished. So I tried to categorize and triage the exhausting list of things I needed to do. Concentrating on and completing one or two things at a time gave me focus and a sense of accomplishment.

Something else that worked for me was finding one positive thing during the day and focusing on that. Often it was a smile or a hug from my children, an hour without thinking of my past, or a day in which my boss found no fault with my work. I realized that if I looked at my day with an open mind, I could find something there to bring one good thought and smile. Then I could focus on that until the next positive thing happened. I wrote these positive thoughts in a journal. On days when I had trouble finding one, I went back and read previous ones.

I wish that during those tough times I had leaned more on God to give me the strength I needed to get through my days, for His guidance and understanding. Eventually, I felt God nudging me to start learning how to live more fully.

CHAPTER 8

GRANDPA'S DYING

"Mom, Dad said Grandpa is a whole lot worse again."

My heart stopped for the dozenth time in the last two years. It seemed I continually had to have my children ready to go to the funeral for their dad's father. Here I go again, brainstorming how to clear their high school calendar of sporting events and school activities. Although it was Tom's father, I knew I would be the one responsible for getting them ready and formulating the logistics for them to travel out of town. One of the children was having a huge acne breakout; Tom would have no patience for this!

I began again making the list I'd made over and over the past months, every time Grandpa's health failed. Do they all need haircuts? Do the boys have suits that fit? Does my daughter have an appropriate dress her size? Do I need to take them out to get the clothes they need?

"What in the world are you doing?" my sister asked. "He hasn't died yet! Why are you planning for something that hasn't happened? You might have to plan it again in six months when they'll need summer clothes instead of winter clothes."

"But I have to make a contingency plan," I offered feebly. "I have to be ready at a moment's notice to take the kids over to Grandpa's house. You know Tom isn't going to help get them ready, but he'll want them to be at Grandpa's house the day after he dies."

Plan, plan, plan. And maybe *this time* it would go well. Maybe *this time* Grandpa will really die. At some point he would die, I figured, so it was better to be ready than become the victim of my abuser's wrath of calling me unprepared and insensitive.

THE LIE: I HAVE TO PLAN, BUT I CAN'T PLAN

There was one thing I could never plan for, and that was Tom's emotional turmoil. All I could do was react. Up to the end of the twenty-one years of my marriage to him, I still couldn't tell when his mood would change. His emotions were as fluid as a watercourse and changed about as often as he blinked.

During the final years of our marriage, each morning I'd stand in the kitchen watching him come down the stairs, begging in my heart that since I had given him that disgusting oral sex he forced me to perform earlier and since I had kept the children quiet, he would give us some temporary peace.

But peace was never what he wanted. He wanted to see me react, stressed out, striving but failing. He loved showing me that he didn't have to do anything to make anything right, but I needed to do everything.

I could only react to him.

When I lived in that world of domestic cruelty, I tried to plan every day and every event so I could perhaps—this once—avoid being yelled at or punished again. But when the day or event arrived, planning never seemed to properly prepare me for what would happen.

For so many abusive years, I blamed myself for not thinking adequately enough. I believed that if I had only reflected on the situation more thoroughly, I wouldn't have upset Tom so much. I needed to get better at figuring things out. I needed to get better at planning.

My imagined timelines always turned out positive results in my head. My plans never matched my abuser's response, but that didn't stop me from trying. This firestorm of planning became second nature to me, even though ultimately every time I simply had to react to the environment Tom created, in the way that benefited Tom, adjusting the situation to fit Tom's needs.

Even though I was now physically separated from my abuser, I still tried to make plans, plans, and more plans to avoid his anger and promises of retaliation. Even though I was separated, I wasted countless hours with great anxiety and spent tremendous amounts of mental energy wondering, second-guessing, and brainstorming all options to "get things right" for my abuser so I wouldn't be the target of his verbal onslaught of obscenities for my "incompetencies" via his phone calls.

My mind was still trained to brainstorm courses of action twenty-four hours a day.

It was a terrible, fumbling mess.

A GLIMMER OF TRUTH

It saddened me greatly to hear from my sister that other people don't continually have to develop so many possible scenarios for everything that may or may not happen in their world. No wonder my head was spinning. I was doing a dance of anticipate, plan-and-react, anticipate, plan-and-react.

But learning that I shouldn't carry on the contingency planning in my head didn't mean I could stop it immediately. It was so much easier for me to just agree with my sister than spill out my fears. Did she really understand what she was asking me to do? Time after time I would agree with her rather than explain my fears.

How would I know when I should plan and when I shouldn't? Was I really supposed to be able to make plans without judging them against how Tom would react? That was a scary thought. My lack of self-confidence convinced me I surely wasn't strong enough to make up such rules while knowing I would open the door to being yelled at more. And what if this time I provoked him enough that he really did kill me?

SEEING TRUTH CLEARLY

After some time had gone by, I began to understand that even in my recovery process I was reacting in crisis mode to almost every situation, because it was the only thought process I knew.

This new understanding strengthened my determination to break down the voices in my head and try my best to retrain my thought processes. I began to see that the problem wasn't really that my life in recovery was just one big walking crisis; it was my *reactions* to the people and events in my world that weren't normal.

Turning the focus away from my abuser and onto my reactions was confusing and difficult at first. But I learned more and more to look to God for guidance about my planning and my reactions. I learned to ask the Holy Spirit for discernment.

It was a challenge learning to separate the voice of the Holy Spirit from the voice of the enemy, the accuser, reminding me of the punishments of my past if I didn't plan and react perfectly.

But slowly and safely, I began looking at my reasons for making the plans I made or reacting the way I did, especially to my abuser's words and actions. I looked deep into my heart and mind to discern my motives.

Eventually I was able to stop brainstorming all possible scenarios and my possible reactions. I began to learn to make sensible action plans and then let the situations that I don't have control over develop without deliberating about them.

MAKING SIMPLE PLANS

In those early days of getting out of the abuse, I called on God for help, leaning on Him for guidance and understanding. I also began to read the Bible regularly.

Beginning to make my own normal plans, proactive rather than reactive, required a huge mindset adjustment. Early in my journey of recovery, I was barely able to plan how I was going to make it to lunchtime. Then when lunchtime arrived, I struggled to plan how I was going to make it to dinner. And then I had to get through the bedtime routine with the children, which was stressful even without Tom around.

Eventually I could extend my planning beyond the next few hours to tomorrow evening. When I started planning the hours in my day, my world felt steadier. I began to feel safer, as I had a better expectation of what was going on.

In the beginning, my planning skills failed more than they succeeded. But I learned that success or failure wasn't really the most important issue. The issue was that I was learning bit by bit to get my life back under control.

I was used to reacting and making contingency plans, which were really just another form of reacting. As I continued to exercise deliberate focus, I refused to continue living in a reactive mode— looking at life through my abuser's eyes—and instead switched to a proactive view of my world, taking action according to the way God wanted me to live.

GOD'S PLANS ARE BETTER THAN MINE

Sometimes along this journey God has asked me to take some action that seemed outside my ability to plan. These have caused intense fear, even when I can see that I'm prepared to do what He is asking, and His timeline has brought me to the point of execution.

When He called me to…

- *leave and stand up to my abuser…*

- *walk through the divorce…*

- *be honest with counselors and doctors…*

- *tell my family members…*

How could I plan for these? How could I get them to work out perfectly? How could I ensure my personal and emotional safety?

I couldn't.

I wasn't ready, I wasn't capable enough, safe enough, or sure enough of myself to be able to follow through on what God wanted me to do. I panicked. Every time.

But every time, when I've finally become willing to focus more on God than the scary and unfamiliar task He's called me to, I've found that I could move forward in God's plan instead of mine. I received the strength and calmness that I needed as I released the final wave of uncertainty and anxiety to Him.

Every time, He has shown me those final pieces of His plan and has replaced my confusion with a sense of peace.

At that moment I know He is empowering me to do what He wants me to do, and my mind becomes overwhelmingly peaceful. He reassures me that regardless of the outcome, my motives and intentions are pleasing to Him.

I can't describe the peace I sense in times like this, but it is the strongest indication for me that I'm doing the right thing. Knowing I'm doing God's will gives me a tranquility that used to be foreign to me. I can calmly complete the task in front of me, knowing that God's strength and loving arms are wrapped around me.

TRUSTING GOD'S PLANS

I used to worry that when I would have to make a big decision I would choose the wrong way and be outside God's will. But if my spiritual growth has shown me one thing, it's that my road isn't a straight one. Lots of curves, hills, and steep mountains fill my journey. Path A might seem like the straight path to get to the result, but maybe it misses some faith-building or character-building experience God wants me to go through, something outside of my ability to "plan" or "react" to, in my vain efforts to try to manage the situation.

God often takes me on detours to make sure I don't miss a valuable learning experience, even sometimes a defeat that will deflate pride and build humility. I need to remember that God wants to develop me by faith into the image of Christ as He walks me through each experience.

I can look back now and say with certainty that the potholes and obstacles God has placed in my path have always developed me into a better Christian, wife, mother, daughter, and coworker.

Romans 12:2 says, *"Do not conform to the pattern of this world, but be transformed by the renewing of your mind. Then you will be able to test and approve what God's will is—his good, pleasing and perfect will."*

God's Word tells me to refuse to conform to the pattern in which my abuser groomed me. It's telling me to break free, with a fresh and exciting mindset closer to the way God thinks.

The years of abuse altered the way I understood my world—my mind was deeply affected. But the mind is also the means through which I receive God's thoughts. How fascinating: the remnants of the abuse and the origin of my faith collide in my mind.

God's strength sits right next to my abuser's stronghold.

It wasn't me and my ability to plan and react that were needed to remove the lingering effects of the abuse from my mind. Instead,

God's grace was required to defeat the stronghold of abuse for me and within me.

When Jesus walked the earth, He released people from the demons that plagued them. After years of hard work and struggles, God released me, tackling and dismantling the thinking patterns that lingered within me from my abusive past.

CHAPTER 9

"YOU LET THE KIDS HEAR YOU ARGUING?"

I remember a conversation with a friend from back when I lived with my abuser.

"What's the matter?" Sherry asked me.

She was just trying to be helpful, I knew, but how could I tell her about the craziness of my world?

"Oh, Tom and I had a fight." I ducked my head a little.

"A fight? What do you mean? What were you fighting about?"

"Oh, it'll sound stupid, really. I didn't fix the steak the way he liked it, and I, um, the different parts of the meal were touching each other, and, well, we just sort of…" my voice trailed off.

"You mean you were yelling at each other?"

"Um…" How could I explain to her that yelling was part of our daily life? How could I explain that Tom was always yelling, and sometimes I yelled back? How could I explain it?

"Wait, you guys weren't arguing like that with the kids home, were you?" she asked pointedly. "That is *so* bad."

I sucked in my breath.

This was one friend who I wasn't going to open up to.

And what a bad mom I was to let my kids hear us when we argued.

I got away as quickly as I could, filled with shame, determined never again to open my world even a crack for others to peek in.

But it happened again, a few years later, when my then-three-year-old daughter's cancer moved to her spinal cord.

"So how's everything?" my friend Lisa asked one day when we bumped into each other at the grocery store.

Should I trust her? *Could* I trust her? But I was in agony and needed so desperately to have someone to talk to.

"Uh…my little girl has cancer…and we just found out it moved to her spinal cord." I was surprised at how quickly the tears jumped to my eyes.

She nodded knowingly. "God is in control," she said, "and He has a plan."

I stared at her dumbfounded.

"He'll carry you through it." She patted me on the shoulder and went on her way.

I watched her go and felt like dissolving on the floor in a sobbing heap. But instead I blinked and turned to the tomatoes.

How can someone speak that way? Cancer was spreading through my child's body for the second time in thirteen months—how could she just glibly tell me everything would be fine?

Maybe everything *would* be fine. But that wasn't what I needed to hear just then. I needed someone to share my pain.

Only one other time did I actually try to talk to someone, only one other time in the twenty-one years of my nightmare existence. It was with a divorced friend, so I hesitantly began to speak about how "challenging" my marriage was becoming. I only barely touched the tip of the horrors.

"Oh, you aren't thinking about divorce, are you?" Sandra's sudden and vehement question took me aback. "It's awful—I speak from experience—and you don't want to do that to your children, no way. You've got to keep your marriage intact. Trust me on this one."

Again, I gazed at her. She wasn't interested in listening either. I turned away.

THE LIE: RELATIONSHIPS ARE TOO DIFFICULT

The people who spoke to me this way thought they knew me. They thought they were dealing with a woman in a normal marriage. They had no idea I was in an abusive marriage, because I was keeping the secret, living in a world of abuse without telling anyone. Inside I was crying out for someone to help me, but all they saw was an overly anxious, even neurotic, woman.

Hurt, shame, and fear all worked against me to convince me that having friends was too difficult. No one would understand. It was easier to withdraw than to get hurt again, or, even worse, to try to explain my awful situation.

My abuser had isolated me, and the few acquaintances I had tried to reach out to didn't understand. When I finally got free of my abuser and started on my survivor's journey, I had few family members and even fewer friends.

At work, especially, I put up my guard, always staying on task, never discussing personal situations, and always looking stoic. I gained the reputation for many years of not caring about others and being a snob.

A GLIMMER OF TRUTH

It was only when I started coming out of my domestic violence cover that I realized I was living a double life, which adversely affected my ability to communicate with the people in my world. Whether it was coworkers, family members, or people at my children's school, the message they gave wasn't always the message I received. They thought they were talking to an average person, yet the person receiving the message (me) wasn't healthy in her thought processes. I didn't hear and see as others imagined I did. I heard and saw through a window of anxiety, fear of personal safety, post-traumatic stress disorder (PTSD), and enormous emotional baggage.

The hardest situations were with family members. As they voiced their concerns about situations in my world, I all too often found myself defending my abuser's actions or inactions because I didn't want them to know the secret terror I lived in. I endlessly justified his words and actions in order to keep someone out who was trying to be helpful. Of course, they were probably correct in their observations of my abuser, but my safety was the bigger fight I was trying to win. Inadvertently, my efforts ended up pushing them away.

When my fiftieth birthday came and only a few family members were there, I knew something wasn't right. I looked back over the previous twenty plus years, at all the relationships I had withdrawn from. Even though I knew I had withdrawn because I didn't want to get hurt, they had no idea why I had done it.

The reason I lost friendships is clear to me now. I had hidden, covered, avoided, and justified so much to so many people. It was easier for me to disconnect with family members and friends rather than explain what was going on in my secret world.

But in the long run, what good was it for me to keep everyone away from me? Who was I hurting here? I was hurting my own ability to let go of my past and be free to move forward with my life.

After many years I knew it was time for an explanation and reconciliation with coworkers. It was a hard task—after all those years of being a stoic, I finally wanted to have real conversations with the people in my life. But it was important to begin crossing that bridge. I knew it was time to begin regaining the ability to talk and listen to others.

CHAPTER 10

FIRST DAY ON THE JOB

I spent hours choosing what I would wear. What would most look like a "power suit"? It was so complicated now that I couldn't just put on my army uniform to go to work.

I was about to go to my first day of my first civilian job after twenty-one years of wearing a uniform.

I knew that from my impressive résumé of army leadership and management they expected me to be a leader among this new college-aged population I'd be working with.

How would I do it? I felt panic rising as I dressed and got the children breakfast. I was no longer wearing the uniform that shielded me from challenges and questions.

Now what did I have to offer them? My decision-making abilities?

The panic rose in my throat as I sat down behind the steering wheel and drove to my new workplace.

I really had no ability to make good decisions, and I knew it. I knew it.

So…I did what I was used to doing. I faked it.

As I stepped out of the car and walked into the building, I switched out my internal struggles with the empowerment of my professional past.

"Good morning!"

I think I sounded bright, cheery, and above all, confident, as I slid behind my new desk.

For the most part, this mask of confidence fooled everyone around me.

For the most part.

I do remember one man asking, "Why are you always apologizing when you didn't do anything wrong?"

Ouch.

THE LIE: MY MASK WILL PROTECT ME FROM MY PAIN

For years, I thought "faking it" was the answer to being able to support myself and my children. I pushed aside my confusion, pain, and anxiety, and instead did my best to exude confidence.

Instead of dealing with my struggles, I minimized them. At some point, I started convincing myself that ignoring my past was the best way for me to move forward.

Although my mask protected me to some extent during those early years, it also served to separate me more and more from reality. I felt like I was faking not only my confidence at work, but also my actions at home. I even got to the place where I felt I was faking being alive.

In the long run, continuing to internalize and deny my painful past rather than facing it caused greater pain and long-term physical and emotional problems.

A GLIMMER OF TRUTH

My sister would say I started my survivor journey as an atheist because I couldn't believe a caring God would have allowed the abuse to happen to my children and me. Yes, there's no denying that I was furious and outraged at God during the early part of my recovery. For thirty days in a row I had prayed, "God, please keep me alive," yet once I was safer, I wandered around aimlessly not knowing what to do next.

But I finally came to a place where I knew that I needed help tackling deep-rooted issues of being able to function in the confusing world outside that "familiar" but toxic one. I was desperate to move on from my situation. I realized there had to be more to my relationship with God than just "keep me alive today." I became desperate to stop simply going through the motions of the day, only reacting to the activities around me, and begin actually living in the moment.

I despised faking being alive and going through the motions of my day. I wanted to know if there was more to life and the reason I was still alive than this.

Eventually I was able to see that God helped other people, but even with all my lack of confidence, I was confident about one thing: He wouldn't help a falling-apart victim like me who couldn't even get her act together.

I didn't even know exactly what I was seeking when I finally turned to Him for help unraveling the mess that my world had become. But I knew He was my only way out; He was my last hope.

Once again, I threw my hands in the air admitting I didn't know what to do to take the next step toward becoming a survivor of domestic violence. At this point, my recovery wasn't a matter of simply surviving versus dying; it became a matter of surviving versus wanting to *be alive*.

As I continued to experience exhausting anxiety and confusion, it became more and more clear that I was unable to recover on my own. I began to beg God for His grace and love. I wanted the internal calmness and peace others were describing. I needed to get out of my confused mind. I wanted someone to save me.

I was perplexed as I had no idea how to find God or, even if I found Him, how to listen for His guidance. And yet, somewhere in the mess of what my world had become, God was still there waiting to help me as soon as I turned to Him. God's patience to walk next to me, nudging me along until I yearned for Him more, is such an amazing gift.

When I started reaching out for God again, I knew He was walking beside me holding my hand. God's support was gentle and kind, prodding me to take practical measures to protect myself from my abuser, not pushing too hard at first.

It is when I found God's love that I felt less like I was simply reacting to my world through my mask but instead responding to my world from my heart.

SEEING TRUTH CLEARLY

But there's a difference between wanting God's help and seeking God as a person. And that is what my relationship with God became, a real, two-way relationship filled with trust, respect, understanding, and love.

As with any relationship, just saying I wanted to be friends didn't automatically make us friends. I needed to invest time and energy in the relationship. That was when I began to see real change.

I found that though I had put the Lord last in my options for help after I had tried everything else, He did not put me last. I found that the more I began to seek Him out, the more I had to thank Him for, and therefore, the more I began to feel His positive influence in my life.

I wish I had genuinely embraced the Lord Jesus Christ and His salvation earlier in my journey. Had I legitimately invited Him into my heart earlier, I would have had a friend and confidant and wouldn't have felt so lonely.

How did I finally surrender to God? I surrendered by inviting the Lord Jesus Christ to come into my life. When I did, He took me where I needed to go. But that meant I had to relinquish the desire to go and do what I wanted. If I genuinely gave God my heart, I was putting my faith and trust in Him, agreeing to go and do what He was asking me.

God's grace, love, mercifulness, and compassion have felt like God's loving arms tightly wrapped around me, protecting me from the evils of my past, yet encouraging me to face the challenges of the moment. Feeling loved by someone again helped so much in filling the void of loneliness from my past.

2 Corinthians 5:17 says, *"Therefore, if anyone is in Christ, the new creation has come: The old is gone, the new is here!"*

I now realize that the Lord has provided me with a remarkable life, one that I could never have imagined possible.

CHAPTER 11

"YOU'LL PAY FOR THIS"

"There is no way in this universe that's going to happen." I slammed the phone down. No way in this universe.

It had been two years since my abuser had left our home after we separated for good. Two long, painful years. And now he wanted to enroll his girlfriend's kids into the same school with my children.

He really thought I'd be fine running into his girlfriend every single day? Who did he think he was?

This phone call was the first time I stood up for myself. And he was planning to make it the last.

"You fuckin idiot." I heard his familiar voice on the voice message. "Who the hell do you think you are talking to me like that? You'll pay for this."

So what did *that* mean? There had been enough times he had hit me with threats, and the one time he had almost killed me. I knew he could hurt me again if he wanted to.

Late that night, near midnight, I heard my ten-year-old son get out of bed and start downstairs.

"What is it? What's wrong?" I asked, feeling edgy.

"I thought I heard somebody at the door, Mom," he said. I followed him as he went to peer out the window beside the door.

As he leaned against the window, the front door flew open and slammed him in the shoulder. He cried out as he was flung back. I cried out. The security alarm blared.

So much noise and commotion yet we never did see who, if anyone, had been at the door.

When the police officer arrived and heard our story, she said, "I don't think I've ever heard about a break-in in this neighborhood before. This is very unusual." Once again, I felt like my heart stopped.

THE LIE: I'LL NEVER FEEL SAFE

Through the years of living with Tom, I had never felt safe because I never knew when his anger would erupt into violence or when he would mutter veiled threats.

Being on constant alert to cater to my abuser's changing moods, demands, and punishments all contributed to my feeling unsafe.

When he almost killed me, I knew I wasn't safe.

Now, even though I was separated from him, how could I ever feel safe?

A GLIMMER OF TRUTH

Years of counseling and growing faith taught me that *being safe* and *feeling safe* are two different things. I knew the importance of precautions that helped me *be safe* and allowed me to be more in charge of my world. I knew that having the house alarm and other safety precautions in place was not paranoia; it was wise, because Tom is a danger.

However, that wasn't necessarily true of other parts of my world.

I remarried and now have a husband who helps me feel safe, but even more, I began learning how to acknowledge my feelings and put safety plans in place.

SEEING TRUTH CLEARLY

My years of counseling helped me to see ways I could help myself *feel* safe. Specifically, I have been able to learn:

- *strategies to feel safe.* For example, prior to entering a crowded area I can remind myself that Tom won't be there, so I can be safe. If I need to, I can ask someone to go with me when I have to be in a crowd.

- *coping skills when I feel unsafe.* I can understand the reasons I feel unsafe in a crowd (people close, loud noises, cigarette smells). I can remind myself that in spite of occasionally being affected by threatening situations, I still have much life to enjoy.

One of the most important things I learned from a counselor—when I was finally willing to go—was about what *triggers* are and how to deal with them.

DEACTIVATING THE TRIGGERS

A trigger is anything that recalls a traumatic experience and brings an adverse reaction. It's anything I see, feel, or experience that takes me back to a painful place from my past.

It sometimes seemed like, after twenty-one years of abuse, my life was filled with one huge trigger after another, sometimes many in one day. Even though I was physically out of the abusive situation, I continued to respond to my world in ways that felt familiar, with little to no regard for how my well-being was affected. I continued to respond to triggers the way my abuser had trained me.

Early on, those triggers gripped me so tightly that the events from the past felt like they were happening all over again. The overwhelming anxiety attacks nearly suffocated me.

I didn't want to relive those painful memories. I didn't want the triggered anxiety attacks.

I needed to learn what my triggers were so I could take appropriate action to deactivate them.

CHANGING THE MUSIC

Something as simple as a song on the radio could take me back to a horrible experience. It didn't matter how quickly I hit the button to change the radio station; it only took a few seconds for the song to disturb my otherwise healthy thought processes.

I countered this trigger by listening to Christian music. Christian music wasn't connected at all to my past, and it gave positive input to my rambling thoughts and filled my mind with encouraging truths.

It also helped me become calmer while driving. In all the things I couldn't control while driving, like traffic, red lights, and whiny kids, I controlled the one thing I could, my music. The louder the music, the less "head noise" I heard.

CHANGING THE DRIVING ROUTINE

Driving generated so many painful triggers for me. I needed to find new routes that didn't go past restaurants, shopping areas, and other reminders of painful events from the past. When the town put up a new billboard that reminded me of one of my brutal beatings, I drove the long way to work for months. No matter how hard I tried to just not look at the billboard, I knew it was there, so I had to avoid the street!

SURVIVING THE HOLIDAYS

When it came to holidays, I needed to identify the celebrations that triggered me because of painful associated memories and plan ahead to counteract them.

And what about the holidays I hated spending alone? I had to decide if it was worth being involved in a family gathering, which could carry its own set of triggers.

CHANGING THE HOUSE

When my children first started going to their dad's house for their weekends, I could have spiraled into depression. Instead, I chose to use that time to give my house a makeover, including painting the interior and beginning the process of disposing of everything that reminded me of my abuser. (I especially never allowed the color from his alma mater anywhere in my house!)

It was more challenging to remove evidence of his physical assaults against me. I painted over scuff marks, or hung pictures or decorations over holes in the wall, but still I knew what was behind the cover-up.

Slowly, though, the ugliness that lay hidden behind some of the things I hung faded in my memory. Over one ugly reminder in my kitchen I have a loving note from my new, kind husband. After all these years, I doubt if he knows what's behind that note.

CHANGING THE MINDSET

Seeing my abuser anywhere at any time was always hard, but at our children's sporting and school events it was incredibly challenging. Sometimes just arriving at the soccer or baseball field where my boys were playing caused me overwhelming anxiety, as I would wonder if my abuser would be there or not. Planning a strategy to get through the event was immensely helpful. Often, I would arrive early or solicit help from someone who would be early, to save me a strategic seat.

Here's another way I planned ahead of time when I knew I would be seeing him: I planned that whatever he did and whatever he said to me at the event, I would hold it *in stasis*. Here's what that looked like:

I proactively scheduled that whatever he would say to me, I would keep it in a mental brown paper bag. It took years of practicing, but eventually, I could drop that brown paper bag into the trash can as I left my child's event. I chose to refuse to allow his hurtful comments to upset me during the drive home and ruin an otherwise fun school event with my children.

Even though I couldn't entirely avoid triggers, I could begin working on minimizing their effects. Identifying them allowed me to start taking small steps to avoid them or counter them, on my journey from domestic violence victim to survivor.

CHAPTER 12

EVENING NAPS

"Mom." My twelve-year-old son was shaking me awake. "Mom, it's time to get up and go back to work."

"OK, baby, I'm coming," I muttered groggily, rubbing my eyes. I looked at the clock. It was 7:00 p.m., and I needed to be back to work in an hour.

I stumbled to the kitchen and hugged myself while the coffeepot gurgled for my nighttime dose of caffeine. "Have you three gotten your homework done?"

"Yes, Mom," they all said.

"What did you eat for dinner?"

"That canned spaghetti you put out for us."

"Oh, that's right." I rubbed my eyes and reached for my largest travel mug.

When my abuser had first noticed me, back when we were both young and he was charming, it was because of how much beer I could hold. But as the daughter of an alcoholic, there was no way I was going to take the chance of subjecting my children to an alcoholic mother. So caffeine had become my drug of choice.

Day after day and night after night I tried to function in this foggy state of mind without entirely realizing what was happening to me. Caffeine woke me up. Caffeine got me through the long day. And when it was finally time to sleep for a few hours at night, sleeping pills did the trick. In addition to working a normal 40 hour a week schedule, two nights a week I went back to work from 8:00– 10:00 p.m. It had been going this way for seven years and was going to continue another three years before my schedule would change.

THE LIE: I'LL NEVER BE A GOOD MOTHER

I had worked so hard to get myself and the children out of a toxic environment and yet, truth be told, my inability to function affected my ability as a mother. I became moody, uninterested, and flat out overwhelmed with every task. I felt stuck, but I had no idea how to get out of the mess that had become my world. My complete ignorance of PTSD and the continued stress I was dealing with robbed me of many mealtime conversations and much enjoyment of my kids. One of my biggest regrets is missing that routine of dinnertime and homework.

Another problem with feeling like a terrible mother resulted from the lack of boundaries between me and my abuser. He continuously analyzed my parenting skills and berated me, often right in front of the children.

You took him to the doctor when you didn't need to.

You should have taken him to the doctor sooner. Now there are going to be so many more problems.

You didn't follow through with the recommendations the way you should have.

When it comes to their health, you can't do anything right.

How could I trust myself to be a good mother when these lies were in my head? It was easier to rationalize being away at my job all the time than have to face my own sense of ineptness when it came to raising my children.

My sense of guilt greatly increased when my oldest son didn't have the grades to get into a four-year college, and he had no particular direction. *"I told you so,"* the voice in my head seemed to say. *"Terrible mother."*

A GLIMMER OF TRUTH

After high school, my son attended the local community college for a year. While he was attending, he found what turned out to be the perfect long-term college for him. In high school, he wouldn't have known to choose this four-year university, but while studying at the community college God helped him become academically confident and aware of this better option.

All this guilt when God's plan was in action! Instead of carrying guilt, I could have been praying that He would fix my regrets with His awesome plans.

SEEING TRUTH CLEARLY

As I began to be able to step back from my heavy burden of guilt and look at my life more objectively, I began to understand some important things.

First, I had lost track of the prime objective of my leaving my abuser: to break the domestic violence cycle. The fact is that if I break that cycle and raise Christian children, then I'm a good mom. God isn't asking me to raise smart or athletic children; He is asking me to raise children who are being taught to be kind and to know Him.

Second, my kids were army kids, moving often and living in domestic violence. This was an uncommon world, but society expected them to function as if it was ordinary. I finally understood that it was okay if my son didn't conform to the typical timelines of his peers.

Third, I needed to set those all-important boundaries with my abuser and then get his voice out of my head before I could even see what being a good mother was all about. I finally saw that the foundation to all good mothering was truly loving my children and providing them with my compassionate support over the long term.

Time proved that all the material gifts their dad provided wasn't what they deeply cared about. My always being there for them, during all the awkward times of growing up, is what they really needed. And that was something that, as I healed, I was learning.

MORE LESSONS TO BE LEARNED

It took me years to acknowledge I was drinking too much caffeine. Eventually I saw that this habit was one thing hindering my progress to recovery, keeping me stuck and unable to move past depression. I needed to understand that just as drugs or alcohol could be unhealthy coping mechanisms, so could caffeine. Finally, I was able to withdraw from my caffeine addiction.

SPEAKING TRUTH: DEPRESSION AND SPIRITUAL WARFARE

In those early days of being out of the abuse, darkness seemed to begin overcoming my days and nights. For the first time, I was trying to get past my years of being told I was stupid, I was worthless, and I couldn't do anything right.

Although I despised it, my abuser had groomed me on how to react to his emotional, physical, and sexual abuse. I had been trained to shut down my thoughts and emotions and simply obey. His abuse brainwashed me so severely that I was unable to think on my own.

Even though I was out of it now, dealing with being a single parent, my daughter's continued health maintenance, financial devastation, having to make decisions on my own for the first time, supporting three hurting children coping with the divorce, and the difficulties my anxiety caused at work…all of it felt like too much.

So many disturbing and confusing thoughts roamed around in my head that finally I began to feel like shutting down was the only thing I could do. I was unable to function in the slightest.

For a long time, I didn't even know I was suffering from depression. That meant I couldn't even acknowledge it was something I needed to work through. As with so many other things, I believed the longer I was divorced and trying to move on with my life, the easier my ability to function would be. But while I kept cycling through the same thinking patterns, I wasn't going to be able to get out. Something had to change.

THE ENEMY'S THOUGHTS IN MY HEAD

I was away from the emotional, physical, and sexual abuse, but I wasn't away from Satan's involvement in the mess of my world, creating continued havoc in my mind with his continued lies. He used those lies to infiltrate my lack of self-worth, trust, and ability to think, worse than I ever could have imagined. Knowing how weak I was, he pounded relentlessly on my indecisiveness.

Given that the devil's main purpose is to spread lies, wreak havoc on human beings, and oppose the truth, my battered mind must have been an inviting playground for him. He didn't have to wait for a particular situation or moment of weakness to inflict chaos. A piece of music, a holiday, a billboard, a birthday, any occasion could be an opportunity for his disruption through accusations, reminders, and lies. He used his lies to manipulate me, discourage me, and turn me anxious, doubtful, and confused.

This confusion and chaos, these lies and manipulations, influenced my interactions with my children, my boss, my sister, and my mother. Doubt became second nature to me, causing a constant firestorm of conflicting emotions every moment I was awake. Any moment I tried to come up with an original idea, those demonic lies were right there waiting to counter my thoughts with second-guessing and self-doubt.

RESISTING THE DEVIL'S ATTACKS

Initially, the devil's distractions came as a surprise. But more and more as I experienced them, I began to cry out to God for help. I began to see that the devil wanted to disrupt my thinking through doubt, frustration, greed, anxiety, or general uncertainty in order to keep me from doing what God wanted me to do.

The Bible states that Satan is an adversary, a strong-willed enemy that attacks us to hinder our advances into God's kingdom. What makes Satan so effective?

He used *chaos and confusion* in my mind, echoing Tom's voice. That was effective for me for years.

He also took advantage of *distractions*. A normal everyday occurrence—the doorbell, the phone, the dryer buzzer, the children squabbling—could pull my attention away from focusing on God.

Besides the chaos and confusion, he also disguised himself, masquerading as *a messenger from God*.

2 Corinthians 11:14 says, *"And no wonder, for Satan himself masquerades as an angel of light."*

Satan might pretend to bring good into my world, but his motives are meant to destroy me or my belief of God. Instead of being a genuine angel of light, a source of positive influence and growth in my world, Satan's true motives are revealed in his desire to spread destruction through sin and deceit. The enemy uses confusion and misdirection much like a magician has us looking in one hand while the coin is in the other.

In fact, as I have tried to remain vigilant and alert, I have also learned to pray for Holy Spirit-led *discernment*. I pray that God will help me recognize the enemy's tricks for what they are. Satan does not want me to advance toward God's will, and I've seen that often his attacks against me increase as I do.

The primary weapon behind each of these tools, though, is *lies*. The way to fight them is with *truth*.

I remember when I was in the beginning stages of writing this book. I woke up at five o'clock one morning excited about the new piece I was going to write.

But as soon as I sat down, I spilled coffee on my laptop, ruining it. At that moment I could have fallen prey to the lies that drew me to the black hole of discouragement, frustration, and even anger. But after that initial moment of panic, I was able to praise God. I knew He would bring me through.

Another time, on the day I started my blog, www.recovering-fromdomesticviolence.com, I also suffered a freak accident that fractured my heel, meaning I would need to use a knee scooter for eight weeks. I could have fallen prey to the lie that I shouldn't try to move forward with this project. Or I could acknowledge that the enemy would love to stop a project meant to help the oppressed and glorify God.

Once I became aware of how Satan works, these tricks no longer fooled me. That's when my life became a bit more interesting. The more I matured spiritually, the more aggressive, subtle, and sophisticated he became in his attacks. He would even do things that were blatantly obvious, bold, and outrageous, and he didn't care if I knew it was him or not.

Always bear in mind that we're at war, in a constant battle of good against evil, and the enemy we fight is not one of flesh and blood. The unpredictability and unexpectedness of Satan's attacks have often reminded me of how my abuse used to unfold.

I can't fight Satan's attacks any better than I could fight my abuser's attacks. But now that my faith is growing, I can cry out to God to fight these battles for me. I can praise Him instead of falling prey to the tactics of the enemy. I can take on the whole armor of God, as described in Ephesians 6, and trust in Jesus Christ to protect me.

As I've been able to do these things more and more, the fog of confusion and depression has lifted.

CHAPTER 13

Too MANY HAPPY PEoPLE

Dressed in a conservative blue suit, stockings, and high heels, I blended in with everybody else.

That was what I kept telling myself, anyway. Maybe they wouldn't notice that I couldn't stop trembling. Hopefully I could keep my overwhelming anxiety internalized and not let the panic show on my face.

Sliding into a seat in the back of the church, I kept my head down—it was just too terrifying to look up. Someone might be looking at me.

I heard two men greet each other boisterously. "Hey, brother! Good to see you, brother!"

I winced.

I peered up quickly to see each of the men returning to their families. Each of them had a happy wife and happy children.

Happy, happy, happy.

It was too much for me.

Singing happy, happy songs.

There was no room for people in pain, like me. People whose lives were messy, like mine.

I felt so alone.

THE LIE: CHURCH IS OVERWHELMING AND LONELY

I can think of few other places where I've felt as alone as I did when I went to a church service by myself. And for that matter, few other places where everyone else seems so perfectly put together and happy. Just the thought of being around so many upbeat people was enough to make wonder if I could achieve my recovery without the assistance of a Sunday morning service.

But I kept going. My mother had been trying to tell me for years that what I needed was a "church family." For twenty-one years I hadn't set foot in a church, partly because I didn't even know who she was talking about when she talked about "God." Was He the God who allowed my abuse? Was He the God who allowed my daughter's cancer? How could He possibly be a God who loved us?

But now, I needed to know who He was, who He really was. I needed something—someone—bigger than myself to set my hopes upon. I needed help in this battle with darkness. I needed to hear music that would encourage me.

I needed church.

A GLIMMER OF TRUTH

One Sunday morning as we were standing to sing, I felt God saying to me, *"Look around at all these people."* I did, and saw more than a thousand pleasant-looking, nicely dressed people.

As usual, they were all happily singing to the music. *What happy lives they all must live,* I thought.

"Don't you remember?" I felt God's Spirit nudging me to truth. *"One out of four of these women has been or will be physically or sexually abused in her lifetime. There's no way you're the only abused women in this building. They're just hiding behind a mask, like you are."*

SEEING TRUTH CLEARLY

When I stuck it out and kept going to the church service, I found other followers of Jesus Christ who could help me know God.

I also found out firsthand that other Christians really do have problems and struggles. Listening to other women's struggles and the painful circumstances they'd navigated with God's help diminished the lie that God had abandoned me.

Listening to sermons from God's Word week after week also became immeasurably instrumental in my life in two ways: increasing my understanding of God's Word and my faith, and breaking the strongholds of Satan's lies in my mind.

Even when I sometimes experienced confusion from a sermon, the experience would eventually propel me to seek the truth to straighten out my confused perspective on my faith. Since I am an auditory learner, hearing God's Word explained greatly helped in countering the abusive thoughts still lingering in my mind from my abuse.

Church doesn't have to be overwhelming. It doesn't have to be lonely. In a good church, the truth will be proclaimed and the people of God will gather and care for each other. This was exactly what I needed in this most difficult time of my life.

CHAPTER 14

MORNING BIBLE READING

So.

Here I was, with my cup of coffee and a large King James Version of the Bible on my lap.

I was ready to get to know God through His Word, seeking His wisdom and guidance.

What a big book. I peered at the paper with the reading schedule I was supposed to follow.

"Morning: one reading from the Old Testament." Okay. I studied the table of contents. Old Testament is at the beginning of the book.

"Evening: one reading from the New Testament." The table of contents confirmed that the New Testament started about two-thirds of the way in.

Okay. Whatever.

I turned to Genesis 1 and began to read, "In the beginning God created the heavens and the earth."

But as I read I had questions. "What is a firmament?" It was long before the days when a word could easily be looked up on my phone.

The language is difficult. Maybe people who've read the Bible all their lives don't have any trouble with it, but I sure do.

I shifted uneasily in my chair but made it through the first two chapters of Genesis.

Evening, it was time to flip to the New Testament and read the first chapter of Matthew. I didn't understand at all why I was supposed to do it this way, but I figured the people who had made the Bible Reading Plan knew what they were doing.

Gah! These names! Who are all these people?

I knew my short-term memory problems would mean I wouldn't retain any of this anyway. I had trouble concentrating in my normal day-to-day activities. Something like this, with its abstract concepts, addressing situations I knew nothing about…well, it seemed pretty pointless.

I'd try again tomorrow.

And try I did. Again and again. I nearly reached the point of giving up.

Thus began my inauspicious adventure in the world of getting to know God's Word. For months, I tried to follow this Bible Reading Plan until I finally gave up; for years I used the difficult-to-understand King James Version, thinking it was the only version available.

THE LIE: THE BIBLE IS TOO HARD TO UNDERSTAND

What I didn't understand then is that there are different levels of "approachability" in the Bible. The Bible is spilt into two parts, the "Old," and the "New." Within those two parts, it contains stories that little children can understand, beautiful poetry, mystical prophecies that scholars still argue over, vital statements of truth about who we are in Jesus Christ, and instructions for how to live in the power of the Holy Spirit.

Those days when I sat by my window with my coffee, I didn't understand any of this.

A GLIMMER OF TRUTH

One Sunday I sat in my newfound church listening to the pastor speak. "I challenge you to read the book of Proverbs three times through this summer," he said. "Read a chapter a day, and you'll cover the book once in June, once in July, and once in August. I believe you'll find that this book will powerfully change your life."

Well, it sounded better than what I'd been doing, so I decided to take him up on it.

Finally, having discovered an easier-to-read version of the Bible (the NIV version), I found that Proverbs was a book that made sense to me. I saw in it descriptions of "the wicked," and I knew I was reading about my abuser. I saw that evil people live as if they have no conscious; trampling over the innocent is what they do.

As I read and understood that bad people do what they do for selfish reasons, this change in my perspective helped me start looking at my abuser differently. I began to consider his evil ways as a reflection of who he was rather than as a reflection of my punishment for past sins. I started honestly thinking that maybe I didn't deserve all that abuse. Perhaps I was a victim of someone else's inability to cope with his world.

The book of Proverbs outlined what happens to those who follow God's wisdom. It was a great place for me to start as it gave me a smorgasbord of little nuggets of wisdom, short verses on how to live and deal with life's circumstances.

Without any self-confidence in how to survive away from my abuser, these verses provided me guidance on how I should live. Without being able to formulate a plan on my own, I found that this book offered me advice on what to do to avoid evil and shelter myself from unnecessary pain.

My counselor had shown me the "Power and Control Wheel" of domestic violence. Now, in the book of Proverbs, I felt as if I was seeing it played out again. I could see that God didn't approve of the selfish and vindictive ways I had been treated. Reading this helped me balance the confusion I felt. I still didn't have the answer to "why" He had allowed it to happen, but I began to be able to better see my situation from God's perspective.

Proverbs has thirty-one chapters, which made it perfect for reading one chapter a day for a month. I did that for three months, just as the pastor had challenged us. Even though I still felt feeble and weak, reading about how I was supposed to respond to these acts of evil provided me hope for how I might be able someday to stand up appropriately.

After three months of Proverbs, I went on to the gospels of John and Luke, eyewitness accounts of the life and work of Jesus Christ. I loved reading how Luke presented the more "human" side of Jesus and John presented the more "divine" side. I was grateful to begin to receive a more thorough understanding of what a true follower of Jesus looked like.

Proverbs gave me guidance on what to do and how to live. The gospels gave me hope that God would love me. Although it still took me years to figure out how to do much of what I need to do, I began to build confidence. Bit by bit I was feeling better prepared.

PART THREE

LIES LEADING UP TO THE NERVOUS BREAKDOWN

CHAPTER 15

NOSY MOTHER

"It's positively ridiculous that he's getting away with that." My mother was fuming about Tom's umpteenth violation of the custody agreement. "Why do you let him?"

"I don't know, Mom." I just wanted her to stop talking about it. "One of the things…"

She barreled on as if she hadn't heard me. "Why are you letting him get away with it?"

"You don't understand what it's like having to deal with him," I began.

"Do you see what he's doing to your children?" She continued her rant. "Do you see this, this, this *obvious* violation, thumbing his nose at you and at the court by taking *your* children across state lines to stay with his *girlfriend*, not his wife, mind you, but his *girlfriend*, when the court order clearly says…"

"I know what the court order says, Mom." I hunched over in my chair, hugging myself. There was no way she would understand.

"He's such a…such a…" She searched for a word. "Jerk isn't good enough. What is he?" She paused. "A cad. That's what we used to call them. Cads."

I sighed. Mom just didn't like Tom because he had taken me away from her. Again that sense of overwhelming loss washed over me. How could she ever understand that?

"So anyway," she continued, "you've got to do something about that cad. You need to take him back to court."

How could anybody understand? How could anybody ever understand the nightmare that had been my life while I was with him, a nightmare that just continued through co-parenting?

The secret fact was that I still feared losing my life. I was still haunted by the image of my children being motherless. Even now I was afraid he could show up at any time and beat me to a bloody pulp if I didn't let him get away with whatever it was he wanted to do. That emotional specter loomed so much larger and stronger than any responsibility I had to my mother.

There was no way I could tell anyone how bad it had been, how bad it still was. That would be crazy. It would be straight-up suicidal.

Surely eventually this nightmare would end, if I could only continue to keep the secret.

"It's going to be fine, Mom. I'll figure out something. I have to get to work in the morning, so I'd better get to bed." I untwisted my balled-up body and shuffled to my room.

THE LIE: I NEED TO KEEP THE SECRET

The fact was I truly thought keeping my lips sealed about the extent of my abuse was the most effective way to keep myself physically and emotionally safe. I kept thinking that if I told, my life and the lives of my children would become even more unsafe. If he knew I had accused him of what he actually did, if he found out I was talking about the abuse…I believed it would be tantamount to asking him to kill me.

I couldn't let the children find out either—I had to try to be the peacemaker in a home that was seething with terror because I wanted their growing up years to be "normal."

My bruises had been documented years earlier, but I still didn't want to let anyone know how bad it had been. Even when I disclosed enough to the doctor so I could get a referral for crisis counseling, I still didn't disclose the full extent of the abuse.

In fact, even though I ended up in specialty clinics over and over again, I never received the proper treatment because I never told the secret. The symptoms were being treated with bandages, when the pain I experienced raged like a cancer.

Even seven years later, "the secret" controlled my thoughts and actions while I remained in relative isolation, hiding behind multiple safety plans. Remaining quiet about the abuse allowed my abuser to trample around in my thoughts day after day for seven years. It brought me uncontrollable anxiety. It brought me another seven years of living but not being alive.

A GLIMMER OF TRUTH

Seven years after I separated from my abuser I experienced a nervous breakdown, the kind of nervous breakdown that stopped my world completely, the kind that scared me into believing I was right back to square one in my inability to function.

But if God hadn't brought my world to a screeching halt with that nervous breakdown, I might never have examined my recovery effort. It brought me to my senses, making it crystal clear that something wasn't right with me.

For a while I had been trying to actively seek out ways to remove the effects of the abuse from within my mind and body. But repeatedly during my recovery effort, the power of the secret hindered my ability to understand what I needed to do and, more importantly, why I needed to be doing certain things.

But now I knew I needed to reassess my current situation. In order for me to learn the coping skills needed to counter the long-term effects of my abuse, I at least needed to be honest with my counselors and doctors.

In order to undo the power of the secret, I had to release parts of it, even a little at a time.

SEEING TRUTH CLEARLY

After a lot of prayers, I knew God was telling me to be honest. I still remember crying hysterically at my sister's house the night before that fateful doctor's appointment when I was going to "tell": I didn't want to share my past with someone who might not keep the information confidential. I was terrified.

But, I also knew God was asking me to tell, so He would be there with me.

Finally, this piece of honesty allowed my physician to correlate my multiple physical ailments with the stress that caused them and get me the assistance and workable treatment plan that I had needed for so long.

It was a rough couple of months, but it was worth it. Finally I had the proper diagnosis and the correct medications, allowing me to:

- deal with the maintenance part of the medicines along with the systemic pain;

- acknowledge my newly diagnosed ailments—including PTSD, irritable bowel syndrome (IBS), teeth grinding, generalized anxiety and depression, and high blood pressure—as genuine battle scars;

⊙   educate myself;

⊙   and perhaps most importantly, take better care of myself so my children did not end up motherless but instead gained a mother who could function.

Breaking the power of the secret was necessary for my recovery and their well-being.

CHAPTER 16

THE WORST PUNISHMENT

Oh, I was having that nightmare again. It always brought back the flashback of that time…that time…

Tom came stumbling into the house way past midnight.

He was obviously drunk.

I was five months pregnant with our third child.

Tom didn't care that I was tired, or that I had to get up early with the two boys, or that I loathed the smell of cigarettes and beer. He didn't care that I hated interacting with him when he was so drunk. All he cared about was that he wanted to have sex. Not loving, intimate, caressing sex, but raw, emotionless, selfish sex. It also didn't matter that sex so late in my pregnancy made me feel very uncomfortable. That was what he wanted: raw, forceful, fighting back the tears, sex.

I'll spare you the details. But in trying to steel myself against the pain, I ended up hurting Tom by accident.

Swiftly and violently I was thrown to the floor, with Tom screaming and swearing at me. I crawled to a corner and curled my legs into a fetal position, trying to protect the baby inside of me.

"You bitch!"

Kick, kick.

"You fucking hurt me!"

Kick, kick.
"Why the fuck.
Did you just.
Do that!
That.
It fucking.
Hurt."
Steady kicks with each word.
"Stay the hell away from me."
"I don't ever want to see your fucking face again! Stay out of my sight!"
Final kick, and then storming out of the bedroom.
But that was only the beginning of what I now know as "the punishment." Three months later, in June 2001, I was scheduled to move to Germany. My three-month punishment for what I had accidentally done that night also meant that—in addition to caring for the house, the yard, and our two boys by myself, which was the norm—I alone would be responsible for all the details of the move.

Any relocation is a headache.

But this was an international move.

With two little children.

When I was eight months pregnant.

And he wouldn't be joining us for several more months which meant I also had to move him into a temporary apartment until he was able to join us.

It was horrific.

THE LIE: I NEED TO KEEP RESPONDING TO HIM QUICKLY AND CORRECTLY OR I'LL BE PUNISHED

Tom punished me plenty of times, but the moving punishment was the worst. For the rest of our marriage, all he had to say was, "You don't want me to punish you again do you?" All the memories of all my punishments, especially that moving punishment, would wash over me again, and I would quickly do whatever he wanted.

Even after we separated, I carried this feeling with me. Even when I rationally knew I was physically safe, still, somehow, it seemed that his superpower capabilities could search out my location in moments. I couldn't get mad at him, even in the privacy of my own locked room. Somehow he would know and punish me.

The control, even from afar, was so complete that sometimes I would even obediently carry out what I knew he would want me to do to avoid another punishment from him. Often it was simple things, like ensuring the boys had haircuts, did their homework, received good grades, finished their chores, or limited their Xbox and computer usage.

The problem wasn't that I was doing these things, the problem was my motive. I was doing these things to avoid being yelled at instead of doing them because they were the right thing to do.

A GLIMMER OF TRUTH

Years after the divorce, I started with a new counselor. When she learned I was still communicating with my abuser, she was shocked.

"You need to stop talking to him," she said.

"Stop talking to him?" That didn't even make sense. We had three children together and lived in the same community. If I didn't answer his phone calls, the voice mail would greet me with a tidal wave of obscenities and hostility. Just seeing his name on caller ID rattled me and filled me with anxiety.

I hadn't said no to anyone in upwards of twenty years. How was I going to start now? And in what fantasyland did my counselor think I could get away with saying no to my abuser…and living to tell about it?

"Stop talking to him and ignore his calls," she said.

SEEING TRUTH CLEARLY

At the same time all this was going on, I was also reading Proverbs. I was getting a foundational understanding of what evil is, how it navigates throughout our world, and what to do when faced with evil thoughts and actions. The book of Proverbs explained to me repeatedly that I cannot change people who invite evil into their world. The best thing I can do to protect my world is to say no and refuse to allow them into my life.

In this way, the Bible reinforced the idea that I can and should exercise my right to say no if I'm being asked or told to do something that will invite evil into my world. I should say no if I'm being asked or told to do something against God's Word and the messages He is placing on my heart.

My counselor explained that it wasn't my job to change anyone. That meant my inability to change my abuser was not my fault! With no power or influence to change other people, the only person I could change was myself.

Even though I couldn't change my abuser's actions or behaviors, I could change my responses to them.

In reality, setting limits on others is a misnomer. We can't do that. What we can do is set limits on our exposure to people who are behaving poorly; we can't change them or make them behave right.

Our model is God. He does not really "set limits" on people to "make them" behave. God sets standards, but he lets people be who they are and then separates himself from them when they misbehave...[2]

When it came to my abuser and his phone calls, learning to refuse them didn't happen overnight. My continued fear of punishment meant it was a slow and painful process.

---

2   Taken from *Boundaries: When to Say Yes, How to Say No to Take Control of Your Life*, by Dr. Henry Cloud and Dr. John Townsend, Copyright Date 2017. Used by permission of Zondervan. www.zondervan.com

But I was determined, and I persevered. First, I ignored every other call. Then I ignored two calls from him before answering. When I deleted his number from my contact list, I was ignoring a phone number rather than a person, a "call from Tom."

Deleting his ability to disrupt my day whenever he felt like it was nerve-racking, but ultimately freeing.

After a year or two, I found the strength to block Tom's number so I couldn't receive texts. Then came the big day when I stopped answering his phone calls altogether. If the call was important, I figured, he would leave a message. If he was just calling to call, he'd hang up. Simple formula!

Easy to say, yet extremely hard to build up the strength to follow through after so many years of conditioning.

What about those times when I absolutely had to talk to him about the kids? If he started getting angry, I could just hang up on him.

In other words, I finally understood that the way to avoid punishment was *not to try to manage his feelings,* but to respond in ways that would keep me safe.

Since he wasn't going to change, I would.

My abuser's ability to control me whenever he felt like it through those terrifying hints of punishment?

I officially took it away from him.

CHAPTER 17

VICTIM IN THE DENTIST'S CHAIR

"Hmm…" The dentist held my x-rays to the light. "Hmm…"

He turned and examined my teeth again, with a gentle tap, tap, tap.

Sitting in the dentist's chair was never easy for me, but this time my anxiety finally bubbled to the top. "What's wrong?" I asked, even though I didn't really want to know.

"I'm wondering about something…" his voice trailed off for a moment. "Is there any possibility you grind your teeth, like when you're asleep?"

"Well, maybe," I replied reluctantly.

"You seem to have loosened three fillings in the past six months." He said it as if I had completed a pretty challenging task. "Do you think it's possible you might grind your teeth that much?"

It had been seven years since I had gotten away from Tom's abuse. Seven years since the last purple and yellow bruise. Seven years since he almost choked me to death.

Seven years of pent-up emotions.

And suddenly all that inner pain that I felt screaming within me came screaming out. "Yes, it's possible! I'm a domestic violence victim!"

But what I meant and what the dentist and dental hygienist heard were two different things. They heard someone who was still in danger. Not only did they offer a free mouth guard for me to wear when I slept, but they wanted to know what they could do to help me get safe.

I sounded like I was still in it. They didn't know I had been out for seven years.

The shame I felt must have turned my face scarlet. As soon as I could I got out of that office so I could drive someplace where they wouldn't see or hear the messy sobs, the inconsolable crying.

THE LIE: I WILL ALWAYS BE A VICTIM

What was wrong with me?

Up until that moment, I have to admit, I had wanted to continue to call myself a victim. It gave me an identity that felt familiar and comfortable, a justification for still being in pain and still feeling kind of crazy. A justification for being afraid to get angry about the abuse.

A GLIMMER OF TRUTH

When I first decided to get out of my situation seven years earlier, my spirit, my faith, my body, and my emotions were battered. Like many other women who attempt to break the cycle, I was tired, miserable, and still juggling all other aspects of my world. My only focus was getting myself and my children away from Tom.

Unfortunately, in addition to having to deal with the physical and emotional effects of the abuse and having to go through the ugliness of a divorce from an abuser, I still had to co-parent with my abuser as well.

The crisis counselor had helped me with understanding why my abuser's actions were inappropriate and why I needed to have a safety plan for myself and my children.

The first long-term counselor helped me understand my situation better and learn coping skills.

But it was the second long-term counselor who taught me about codependency, and even more important, boundaries. The first boundary she helped me implement was blocking my abuser's phone calls.

SEEING TRUTH CLEARLY

My counselor told me to read *Boundaries: When To Say Yes, How To Say No,* by Dr. Henry Cloud and Dr. John Townsend. That book, which provides a precise explanation of God's guidance on boundaries and how to establish them, delivered revolutionary truth to me. My abuser had violated every boundary I had, including my self-respect, self-worth, and self-confidence. The thought of establishing boundaries with him, even seven years out, seemed overwhelming and confusing.

With my therapist's help I began to plan my boundaries, those invisible fences to help me be and feel safe, especially to guard against my abuser and all the fiery darts the devil threw at me through him.

For the first time after my nervous breakdown, seven years into my recovery, I also began taking a serious look at other people in my world and how interacting with them affected me. For the first time I established a safety zone of who I allowed to get close to me and who I didn't, according to whether they intended good or ill. If those who intended ill toward me were offended, I had to learn to let go of the responsibility for their negative feelings that might result from my newfound boundaries.

I had to sort out whether the people in my life were just aggravating (which meant I needed to work through my self-centered concerns), or whether they intended to harm me. Sometimes I needed guidance to see which was which.

While my therapist and I were brainstorming strategies for my boundaries, I continuously sought God's strength and guidance, through prayer and the Scriptures. Then, when I felt God's peace surrounding me, I acted on establishing limits regarding who I allowed close to me. It soon became apparent that I was trying to fulfill my Christian duties with little regard to how my actions were affecting me.

Setting physical boundaries of personal space can be very challenging and sometimes even dangerous. But I found that as I began to acquire little islands of safe spaces, I began to heal and grow in my self-worth. If I didn't sense His peace regarding a decision I was about to undertake, I aborted the plan. It gradually became easier and more natural to establish appropriate boundaries.

As I developed boundaries for my physical safety, I realized I needed them for emotional safety as well. Allowing no evil beyond the boundaries of my safety limits was a huge mental shift in my thinking and took many months of constant, deliberate effort. I knew it was a spiritual battle too, because the enemy would love nothing better than for me to have weak boundaries against evil.

Even though there were plenty of mistakes along the way, plenty of times when my boundaries were violated, eventually, refusing to allow my abuser (or other destructive people) to assault my boundaries increased my peace and calmness, decreased my anxiety, and brought stability to my life.

Romans 8 tells me to "walk in the Spirit," with my thoughts, actions, and reactions under the control of the Spirit of God. My human nature, on the other hand, causes me to feel responsible for other people's thoughts, actions, and reactions.

Setting boundaries has for me been about establishing self-control over my actions, and most importantly, my *reactions* toward others' words and actions.

Switching from a human perspective to a spiritual perspective has been tough. It has required intense self-control and prayer to set my heart right. But, my effort has paid off. Establishing my boundaries has been a critical tool in defeating my abuser's impact on my world.

And it has helped me shed the label "victim" for good.

CHAPTER 18

BANKRUPTCY COURT

I gripped the steering wheel, staring straight ahead, not seeing the sunny morning and clear blue sky. Bankruptcy court was forty-five minutes away, and soon after arriving there I was going to lose my house.

When we were married, Tom had wiped out our entire life savings putting down payments on rental properties.

I knew we were borrowing too much for such a volatile investment. But like all other aspects of Tom's world, my opinion and cautious comments had been totally ignored.

Now, a couple of years after the divorce, Tom's rentals were failing. I was numb.

Due to Tom's mismanagement of our life savings, I was about to lose the house in which I was raising our children.

My thoughts couldn't function. I was unable to fathom the impact of what was about to happen. I felt a churning in my stomach like I would throw up any second.

It seemed that Tom had taken everything from me. My mind, my spirit, my ability to enjoy my world. Now he was taking away the means to raise my children comfortably. If I lost this house, I wouldn't be able to replace it.

I couldn't process all these crazy, swirling emotions.

But obviously, I couldn't get mad at him. What would that accomplish? Another verbal assault on my vulnerable worth?

Or even more confusing, a harsh verbal assault on how this really was my fault even though I never wanted those rentals in the first place?

Sitting in the car outside the courthouse, I knew I couldn't get mad. I couldn't voice any of the swirling feelings of pain, anger, and resentment. I was about to be forced out of my house and I felt overcome with embarrassment and shame. Where would the trail of my horrible failed marriage end?

But as quickly as these thoughts entered my consciousness, I shut them down, telling myself there was nothing to be gained from turning emotional about this. So the only emotion I allowed in was to "be strong."

"Be strong" for the assault from bankruptcy court that was about to happen. Put on my mask of strength and "be strong," not only for the shameful situation I was about to face, but for the enormous moving task I would have to undertake soon after.

Just "be strong," I told myself, and I could get through this. If I allowed one emotion besides "be strong" into my thoughts, I probably would have fallen apart emotionally.

And there was no way I could let that happen. After all, I told myself with a shrug, my feelings didn't matter. I just needed to "be strong."

THE LIE: I JUST NEED TO BE STRONG

I didn't know it at the time, but the *emotional numbness* I felt was a common symptom of PTSD. I called it "being strong," but really it was an inability to cope with the enormity of the trauma being heaped upon me.

When I finally went through counseling, I learned the symptoms of PTSD. Well, what do you know, they fit me like a glove.

Challenges concentrating. Check.

Lack of short-term memory. Check.

Feelings of detachment from my surroundings. Check.

Needing to avoid crowds. Yes.

Racing thoughts. Oh yes.

Overwhelming anxiety. Yes, even to the point that reading, understanding, and questioning are still difficult for me.

But I thought all these problems would pass as I continued to "be strong." I didn't know there was anything I needed to know.

A GLIMMER OF TRUTH

I now realize two important truths about PTSD. First, continued stress prohibits the brain from returning to a normal state of functioning, which eventually alters its ability to function. The mental challenges I continue to deal with as a result of the trauma I endured are the biggest obstacles I face daily. And second, as stress continues and intensifies over time, physical ailments can result, sometimes permanently. I may have ignored a few of the side effects of my PTSD, but when I had to start taking medication for high blood pressure, my attention quickly changed.

SEEING TRUTH CLEARLY

One of the most important tools in my healing journey from trauma and its effects is spending daily time with God, in prayer and reading.

I can't overstate how important this has been to me. Like any other relationship, the more time I devote to its development, the stronger the relationship has become.

STARTING IN THE MORNING

Since I am a morning person, I start each day in the early morning quiet, when there are no distractions, by sitting in the same place, opening my thoughts and prayers to my Father God, for His peace and calmness. My two little dogs realize that when I sit in this place on the couch there's no playing with their toys or getting me to pat them. They curl up next to me and know that after the devotion is when they can start their day.

READING

I enjoy reading a daily devotional and prefer a printed book, as anything electronic distracts me and allows my eyes to wander. An old-fashioned book, one that I can write in and carry with me, has worked best for me. Since my memory is short and I continue to be a new learner, I often read the same devotional years apart. I'm now rereading one from five years ago. It is amazing how differently the words impact me in just a short time in my spiritual growth.

PRAYING

When I pray, I always start with huge thanks for who God is and what He has done in my life or what He is about to do. I am indeed thankful for all that God has done for me. Then I tell God about my confusion, my pain, and the highlights and low points of my day, talking to Him about everything that is important to me.

When I make requests, I try not to limit God. For example, to pray something like, "God, please bless me with the job I'm interviewing for today! I want to work here!" sounds like I know what's best for me and it's God's role to bless me with my desires. Instead, if I'm unhappy in my current job, I can pray for God's intervention to first show me if my desire to change jobs is in line with His desires for me, and if it is, to provide me with a job that is a better fit for me.

Asking God to provide the best answer to my prayers allows for me to see the great and awesome ways that He blesses my world. Just because my prayers are not answered in the way I want doesn't mean that it won't work out; I find God's way of answering my prayers so much more exciting than I ever could have imagined!

TALKING TO GOD THROUGHOUT THE DAY

I also talk to God throughout my day; it seems I'm constantly in conversation with Him about something or other.

This is a learned trait for me, since I didn't grow up with the concept. It was such an unknown. And besides, I was used to constantly rehashing the devil's negativity in my head. I could go around and around in my head in an endless conversation with the devil when he wanted to rile me up and distract me, yet my initial conversations with God seemed so hard.

How could it be so easy to continue the debilitating conversations with the devil, but so hard to just have normal conversations with God? The strangeness of this struggle almost made me want to laugh.

But I knew I couldn't hear God if my head was spinning and my thoughts flying around. I needed to deliberately discipline my thoughts. It has required a lot of mental redirection, but I've learned that turning away from the negativity and embracing positive, faith-based thoughts is so much healthier for me.

At the start of a negative thought, the devil's "comments" on the situation, I purposely push that it aside and replace it with talking with God. As I became more and more used to doing it, it became much easier.

Yes, talking to God is different than listening to the devil's take on a situation, and it is so much better for my ability to stay emotionally confident!

THE END OF THE BANKRUPTCY STORY

My abuser caused untold chaos, destruction, and loss in my life and the lives of our children. I entered that courtroom thinking "be strong."

Be strong and the day will eventually end.

Be strong and eventually the kids and I will move someplace and get this behind us.

Be strong and this whole embarrassing situation will just go away.

Yet God had a different plan for that day. Just before the judge came out, I was called to a conference room.

It seemed there had been a mistake in the calculation on one of the forms. My lawyer apologized for the oversight.

The house wasn't being taken away from me. I was free to go.

Gazing out the car window, I could see the sun shining against the clear blue sky. I will forever remember how colorful the scenery looked that day.

The forty-five-minute drive home was drastically different from the drive to the courthouse. As I praised God for what He had just done for me, it was the first time in years I had truly smiled.

CHAPTER 19

ACCIDENT ON THE HIGHWAY

"Everybody buckled?"

"Yes, Mom!"

"Okay, let's go!"

I got behind the steering wheel feeling the happiest I'd felt since Tom and I separated three years earlier.

"I can't wait for pictures at Grandma's house," I said as we drove.

"I love my dress." My eight-year-old daughter smoothed the ruffles of the adorable purple flowered dress I'd found for her. I glanced in the mirror at the two boys looking spiffy with their new haircuts.

"Yes, we're going to look good in these pictures," I muttered again triumphantly. The six-hour drive to my mother's house for Easter weekend wasn't too big a price to pay to prove what a happy, well-put-together family we were.

See? Time was passing, and we were recovering. We really were. I smiled.

I knew it might take years to recover fully from something that had taken years to happen, but I could see I was getting better. That adorable dress and those cute button-down shirts just proved it.

Two hours into the drive we passed the exit where Tom's parents lived, where Tom would be for Easter weekend. I quelled the familiar anxiety and kept my eyes on the road.

An hour later, our plans suddenly changed.

Everything about that day changed.

When I slowed down for traffic, the semitruck behind me didn't, and rear-ended our van.

"Are you okay, is everybody okay?" I cried out.

"Yes, Mom," said my two youngest.

But the oldest, who had been sitting in the very back, held his shoulder, where the seatbelt had been restraining him. "It hurts," he said. "But I think it's okay."

The police arrived and did the paperwork. My van was drivable, at least.

I tried to corral my swirling thoughts to figure out what to do.

Should I turn around and go back an hour, so Tom and his parents could look at my son's shoulder?

Or should I keep going to my mother's house and figure out what to do then?

I couldn't stand to think of seeing Tom, so with my stomach churning, I kept going.

But as I continued to drive, it was hard to focus on the weekend or the road or even my children's needs. All I could think about was how Tom was going to respond when he heard this news. As if being rear-ended by a semitruck wasn't bad enough, I knew there was no way I handled this situation the way Tom wanted me to.

The way Tom wanted me to.

Even though we'd been separated for three years.

Over the next three hours driving to my mother's house, I felt the anxiety rising and rising. *I should turn back and go to Tom's parents. I'm going to get yelled at anyway. I might as well get it started now.*

No. Deep breath. Keep going.

As I approached my mother's, I could feel the anxiety taking over all of my body. I was shaking. I could barely breathe.

By the time we arrived, my son seemed fine. My parents confirmed it. I could breathe again, finally.

We had a happy Easter and even took those pictures. I tried not to think about the verbal assault I knew was coming.

And come it did.

Even after three years, just seeing his name on the caller ID caused my anxiety to quadruple. For days Tom verbally assaulted me for being "such an idiot" in the way I had handled the accident.

But surely, with the passing of time, all these things would get better.

THE LIE: I'LL GET BETTER AS TIME PASSES

For so many years, I tried to convince myself that the longer I was away from my abuser, the easier my situation would get, the clearer my thinking would be, and the fewer strange symptoms I would have.

When I had a nervous breakdown seven years after getting out of the abuse, this complete collapse served as a serious wake-up call for me. Obviously, what I'd been doing for seven years wasn't working. I was going to have to take concrete steps to get the remnants of my past out of my body and mind. Something was terribly wrong.

Time alone wasn't going to get the job done. Denial wasn't working anymore.

Where was my recovery going, anyway? Distancing myself from my past wasn't the best way to get over my pain? Who knew?

How could I strengthen my thought processes? Could I even recover, ever?

After the fog from the breakdown cleared, I dove back deep into figuring out my recovery strategy.

This time I was going to face my inner self. Reluctantly, I decided I should go back into counseling, and this time I was going to be honest.

A GLIMMER OF TRUTH

Not only did I have to address the aftereffects of the abuse that the medical community could help with, but I also had to face the fact that my way of dealing with things had not worked.

Could I battle the ongoing confusion in my thoughts?

What would happen if I took a stronger stand against the random, harmful memories in my head? Would this even be possible?

I hated having to admit that my life had been so horrible that it was creating such a battle. It made me feel even more violated to have to acknowledge it, even more separated from the world I was trying to adjust to.

At first the situation seemed too much for me to challenge, which meant for a time, darkness returned to my world. But this self-pity mode (that's what I've come to call it) didn't last too long this time, because I knew from my previous seven years, allowing myself to be overcome by the pain didn't help. Regardless of how significant I thought my efforts had been at removing my abuser from my world, experience taught me that looking backward in my recovery efforts never worked to my advantage.

SEEING TRUTH CLEARLY

Now that I decided to lead with more honesty, counseling proved to be more efficient.

Yes, it was painfully hard to admit that seven years out of the abuse, I still viewed my world as completely vulnerable to my abuser's attacks.

And it was worse to admit that the "attacks" weren't necessarily even something he was currently doing but were simply remnants of the thoughts in my head, reactions to something that had or hadn't happened in my world.

My abuser didn't even have to be around to cause me anxiety; my trained mind just continued to race in circles responding as he had taught me. Even without being present, Tom was still controlling my thinking.

I had to set the stage for an incredible battle: the fight for my mind. I had to battle to be alive here within the moment, to be consciously aware of where I was and how the environment was affecting me. This wasn't something I could look at later; no, I had to address these random thoughts immediately, as soon as they occurred.

In addition to the weekly counseling sessions, I focused my efforts on learning to analyze the voices in my head. I began planning to create changes in my life. Slowly, I began to be able to walk in truth.

CHAPTER 20

WHITE BASEBALL PANTS

"You can do it! Go! Go!" I stood up in the bleachers and cheered my son as he stole another base.

"I knew you could do it," I whispered under my breath.

But my smile of motherly pride froze as I watched him slide in the dark red clay, the stripe of mud spreading from the knee to the ankle, thick, heavy, and wet.

Curse those white baseball pants. My head pounded and I could hardly even enjoy the rest of the game. I was going to have to spend hours in the laundry room yet again, scrubbing and bleaching those pants until they were spotless.

For eight years, from the time he was nine until he graduated from high school, I loved watching my son play baseball. Yet I hated cleaning his game uniforms. Despised it.

My abuser grew up playing baseball, so of course he was the expert in how to make sure our son looked the way he should on the field: uniform with no stains, ever. (Now of course, Tom didn't ever take it upon himself to make sure his guidelines were fulfilled. That was completely up to me.)

Back home, after my son stripped out of his filthy uniform, I got to work rinsing, soaking, scrubbing, bleaching and re-bleaching, not just the pants—though they were the worst—but the entire uniform. Under my breath I muttered, jealous of the moms whose sons got to wear gray or blue pants. Oh, how I wanted such a simple gift in my chaotic world.

I was taught that dirty pants meant I was lazy. Dirty pants would embarrass our son. Dirty pants meant I wasn't a caring mom.

Season after season for eight full years I stressed over my son's white playing pants. What if another mom noticed the stains? She would realize what a crappy mother I was. Or I knew my son would be so embarrassed. (Years later he would laugh at me for really believing this was true!)

One evening, though, I sat on the bleachers as usual, watching my son, now a junior in high school and going on his seventh year of baseball.

For some reason, for the first time, I noticed something. I noticed that the uniform the pitcher was wearing had dirt on the knee—dirt that I knew was from last night's game.

His mom sat near me, so I leaned over to her and said lightly, "I'm envious of you, letting your son play with yesterday's 'sliding' dirt still on his knees! I wish I could do that."

The mom looked confused. "Well, of course," she replied. "I don't even wash his uniforms. If he wants them cleaned, he does it himself."

Wait, what? I stammered out a question. "What about the rule of clean pants?"

"The rule of clean pants?" She looked genuinely puzzled, as if she had never heard of it.

"You know, today's uniform can never have any of yesterday's dirt on it."

"Oh, no, no, no," she replied vehemently. "Just look at all the players. Look at all their uniforms. All of them have ground-in dirt!"

Somehow, when I looked around at the players that spring evening, I felt as if my eyes were opening for the first time. For the first time I saw, yes, she was right. Many of the players' pants were muddy. "It's nearly impossible to keep white pants clean, you know," she went on, "especially this late in the season."

Didn't I know it. Every year as the season progressed it had required more hours in the laundry room.

But as her words rang in my ears, and my eyes opened to see what the other players actually looked like, something in my mind opened too.

All these years, even after leaving my abuser, I had been cleaning my son's pants for the wrong reasons.

I didn't want Tom to yell at me if he saw our son's dirty pants. *Yes, that one had been true in the past, but I wasn't even around Tom anymore.*

I didn't want other mothers to see what a terrible mother I was. *But...obviously, this one didn't matter. The other mom pointed out the evidence herself.*

My abuser's voice in my head was still telling me I needed to do it. *Oh...that was it.*

Situations like this one caused me to stop and reassess the conflicting thoughts in my mind. What else did I think were my own thoughts that were really Tom's thoughts "implanted" in me?

THE LIE: I'LL NEVER BE ABLE TO DISTINGUISH MY OWN THOUGHTS FROM HIS BRAINWASHING THOUGHTS

When I began to accept the realization that the thoughts in my head weren't even mine, words can't describe the depression that set in. Imagine coming to the realization that after being told for twenty-one-plus years to "just deal with it," "don't talk back to me," "your opinion doesn't matter," and all sorts of other degrading comments, that I had lost my ability to think on my own. I had to open the denial door some more and realize that there was a huge possibility that Tom had brainwashed me.

Here I was, seven years removed from my abuser, and somehow he still controlled my thoughts, which strongly influenced my actions.

I felt as if I were a puppet whose controller held a remote. My abuser didn't even have to do anything anymore to cause me confusion. After all those years with him, my view of the world and how I processed it was so damaged that he didn't even need to interact with me anymore.

It was a long, sad season when I realized that through his twenty years of emotional and physical battering Tom had changed my thought processes so much that he was still controlling me.

A GLIMMER OF TRUTH

The battle for control of my mind had begun, but it is ongoing. The difference between then and now, though, is that I have learned to minimize the negative influences and strengthen the positive ones.

As I started to listen to the voices in my head, the rhythm sounded like a three-way tug of war. As I started breaking down the voices, the three prominent ones appeared to be:

- my abuser's thoughts and commands,

- my selfish humanness (called "flesh" in the Bible),

- my Spirit-led self following God's Word and the Holy Spirit.

I called this the Me-Myself-and-I battle in my head.

Again, with no guidance, I invented a way to distinguish what I was listening to. I had to be able to recognize the voices before I could figure out how to deal with them.

When I started on this experiment, all I knew was that all three voices managed to keep my head spinning for years. Without any rest, my thoughts were a tangled mess of whatever my fatigued state focused on at the current moment.

Tom's psychological warfare surely seemed the strongest of the three voices. The memories of my abuse heard in his voice seemed perfectly normal, leading the way in convincing me what to do, when to do it, and why it was the right thing to do.

I began breaking down the motivation of each thought:

Me: Being "Me" involved doing things totally focused on my abuser, including what he used to tell me, what he would think is best for him, and my human emotions of greed, lust, and revenge.

Myself: Being "Myself" involved doing things that I thought were best for myself, mostly focused on selfish goals and selfish motivations.

I: Being "I" involved doing thing's God's way according to Jesus' example and the Bible.

In addition to focusing on my *thoughts*, I also started focusing on the *feelings* the idea provided to me. Thoughts left over from my abusive past all seemed destructive to my well-being. They focused on what benefited my abuser; they sounded like my abuser; they were negatively repetitious and countered the positive changes I was trying to make in my life.

My own voice in the equation (it was interesting to observe that I still had a voice) mostly supported the goal that I was working on at the time. My voice was weaker than my abuser's, but when I listened, it moved me forward positively, emotionally, and toward physical safety.

Views from faith provide calmness and peace.

SEEING TRUTH CLEARLY

GOD'S STRENGTH

When I couldn't find the strength to do what needed to be done, God within me (the Holy Spirit) provided me with the strength to do the hard tasks.

I didn't have to rely on my waffling, anxious capabilities; instead, God stepped in with His mighty strength and took over completing the challenging tasks for me.

God's power provides me with the confidence and strength to do what is right, or the calmness to get through the situation at hand.

Philippians 4:13 says, *"I can do all this through him who gives me strength."*

What does this mean to me, a lonely domestic violence victim?

It means that with God's strength, I am strong enough and powerful enough to defeat my enemy's tactics and attempts to disrupt my world.

This verse means that I can defeat all my abuser's advances, those stronghold reminders in my mind and those he surprises me with day to day.

God's Word promises to restore and strengthen all of me, with no pieces left to harm me anymore. The catch is that it is all by faith. I must follow His leading.

PASSION VERSUS DISCIPLINE

Many people are passionate about something. Let's say one of my sons is excited about playing football. If he never practices on his own time, never conditions his body during the offseason, never devotes hours to watching the greats on television, his passion won't make him a great player.

It's the people who act on their passions through discipline, preparing their minds and hearts twenty-four hours a day, seven days a week, who bring their passions to fruition.

When my abuser left me, I had a passion for being a great mom and breaking the domestic violence cycle. I wanted to replace my tired, stressed-out, snapping, and disciplinary tone with a compassionate, loving environment.

My abuser's departure alleviated major stressors in my world, but others seemed to take their place.

For the longest time, my mentality was still in a vulnerable, easily shattered state. I always knew I was breaking the cycle for my children, but for the longest time knowing I was doing it for them was the only thing that defined by my willpower.

It wasn't until I decided to discipline my thoughts and actions—a deliberate act of mental and physical willpower—that I obtained my desired state of being a better mom.

I had to act on my desire (passion) to be a better mom twenty-four hours a day, seven days a week, for years and years.

I had to become personally connected to my thoughts, motives, and actions.

To do this, I had to stop continuously to analyze what I was thinking and why I was thinking it. I had to become personally involved in my entire thought process. Not just sometimes, not just on Sunday mornings or after significant counseling sessions, but all the time.

Since I was the only one aware of what I was thinking, I found it easy to convince myself that I was doing the right thing. If asked, I could always figure out the right answer to convince others (or myself) that I was in control of my thoughts and actions.

But, what did God see in my heart? What did God hear in my mind?

I had to work on the thoughts and motives God could see, not those that I convinced myself existed.

Passion without action can be a great feeling. But passion combined with discipline can produce tremendous changes, and together they enabled me to achieve my goal.

I couldn't adjust my thought processes utilizing my human abilities; I had to bolster God's discipline within me to make these significant and powerful changes in my thought patterns.

For me, becoming spiritually trained required maturity in my spirit and mind. It involved being deliberate in two practices:

- delayed gratification—doing the hard work now so that I can enjoy the rewards later;

- advanced decision-making—determining what action will glorify God and choosing that option.

Merriam-Webster defines discipline as "a way of behaving that shows a willingness to obey rules or orders."

Simply stated, being disciplined is doing what I know will bring glory to God regardless of my feelings or circumstances.

For me to become more disciplined in my words and actions, I had to stop making deals with the devil (otherwise known as my abuser's influence in my head) and build a stronger alliance with God. I had to let God's will and God's way be the deciding reasons on why I acted or didn't act.

Finding the discipline I needed required extreme self-control; sometimes, it was painfully hard. But there is one thing I have learned to believe: control of my thoughts and actions is one of the strongest characteristics that will get me out of the victim world and closer to the survivor world with God.

For me to be able to do the hard tasks that require enormous discipline, I learned and practiced praying for and leaning on Him for His strength and guidance.

During the early phases of my recovery, I learned a valuable lesson about discipline. I finally understood that discipline is not a passion, desire, or want; it is an act of willpower.

For me to get through my recovery and closer to becoming a true survivor, I had to focus explicitly on my ability to discipline my thoughts and words according to God's will and guidance.

Hebrews 12:11 says, *"No discipline seems pleasant at the time, but painful. Later on, however, it produces a harvest of righteousness and peace for those who have been trained by it."*

How did I work on becoming more disciplined?

I worked on training just like an athlete who wants to make it to the next level.

Serious athletes train daily, polishing their skills, but also focusing on what needs to be improved.

I went back to the basic principles I talk about throughout this book.

I immersed myself in the skills, beliefs, thoughts, and actions I felt comfortable with and dug deeper into what would make me a better disciple for God.

Following God at this point meant that I could honestly say, "I care more about what He thought" than what I thought or felt.

Every small victory God gave me, I returned with praise for Him.

Outwardly giving praise to God and offering Him my changed heart seemed to be all that He was asking me while He equipped me to face my Goliath.

Satan's spiritual warfare increased threefold against me during these times of taking a stand against evil.

His schemes were devious and often hard to decipher if I took my focus off identifying the voices in my head.

During this time, Satan used a powerful weapon of doubt to attack me.

He bombarded me with false thoughts of what a waste of time this all was since God didn't love me.

Or what I believe to be Satan's favorite tactic: God's not answering my prayers because I am not worthy.

It is only through God's strength within me that I could break down the huge battle in my mind for control of my thoughts.

After spending so many years reacting to my abuser's control, it was unbelievably hard to gather up the strength to fight him, even if the fighting was in my head and not directed at him personally.

Often, the argument seemed so one-sided: my abuser had the devil's strong, disruptive support.

But the more I learned how to leverage God's strength to counter the evil thoughts in my head, the easier it was to stand up for control of my mind.

CHAPTER 21

THE GUILTING SERMON

"Don't you see," the pastor was saying, "that He always cares for you? We do Him such a disservice when we don't trust Him, when we worry, when we're anxious. We can go to Him with everything that's on our hearts.... "

The pastor kept talking, but I couldn't hear anything else. I felt so anxious it seemed like my eardrums would burst.

Of course, he was preaching on that verse of Philippians 4:6, *"Do not be anxious about anything, but in every situation, by prayer and petition, with thanksgiving, present your requests to God."*

After all the work I'd done, was I going to be rejected based on a technicality? I had to take medicine because I was an anxious person. I had tried to get off it but couldn't. Did that make me a lesser Christian, or no Christian at all?

My stomach churned as our pastor droned on. If what he was saying were true, then I supposed I didn't even belong in God's kingdom. I wasn't welcome in God's world. Panic rose higher.

I had been through what seemed like unbearable pain. During the last two years living with my abuser, my father died of liver failure days after I was promoted to lieutenant colonel. Four months after my father's death, my daughter was diagnosed with leukemia; twelve months later, her cancer spread to her spinal cord which required a bone marrow transplant to save her life. Four months after my daughter's transplant, while she was still struggling on twenty-five doses of medicine a day to survive, my mom suffered a life-threatening stroke.

Was God going to condemn me for being anxious in the face of these horrific events in my past years? Now, on top of anxiety, I had guilt and confusion. Could I have any kind of relationship with God at all?

If it hadn't been for the Christian counselor I was meeting with, this might have been the last church service I attended.

THE LIE: "ANXIOUS PERSON" IS MY IDENTITY

During the early months of my separation from my abuser, I thought my anxious feelings were directly connected to him and all the painful things going on in my world. I believed that as soon as I got through the divorce proceedings and time went by, my anxious feelings would go away.

But now several years had passed, and my anxiety hadn't gone away. In fact, it seemed worse.

I had been anxious when I was living in the abuse, of course, but still, back then I was always able to function. Somehow my abuser's constant demands and unpredictability kept me constantly on the move, trying to make him happy.

But the anxiety I was feeling now was different. At times, I felt more overwhelmed than I ever had. I felt incapable of thinking, focusing, making decisions, or functioning as a mother, daughter, or coworker. It overpowered me, debilitating me much of the time.

Finally, I came to the conclusion, "I'm just an anxious person." It made sense. It was part of my identity. It was who I was. Anxiety had taken over so many pieces of my being that I comfortably found refuge in accepting this title as my identity.

An even worse thought during those years was this: I believed my anxiety was the source of my will to fight. I believed my anxiety was the lifeline of my inner strength. For many years, I thought of my anxiety as a meter or gauge that guided me to decide if I should fight or run. In the absence of any other decision-making method, I let my level of anxiety dictate how I handled a situation.

Mysterious physical ailments began to cause pain throughout my body, but I never connected them to the anxiety I constantly experienced. For some strange reason I just didn't seem to be able to move forward toward a complete recovery.

A GLIMMER OF TRUTH

"Anxious person" makes a very unhealthy identity, and one that would have killed me if I had allowed it to continue. Rather than being an identity, I had to switch my anxiety into a clinical diagnosis. The anxiety I had and was experiencing was a battle wound from my abuse.

But it took a long time to understand this, so long that my health did become endangered.

By this time I had been to over fifty counseling sessions, with a crisis counselor and multiple professional therapists. Yes, these professionals had taught me better ways to cope and prescribed me medication.

For a long time, I have to admit, I believed my anti-anxiety medicine indicated a lack in the "be anxious for nothing" department. Was I weak because I couldn't give my anxiety to God? Was I less of a Christian because I needed this medication? As the daughter of an alcoholic, was I trading one addiction for another?

But I learned that my medication helped restore a chemical imbalance in my brain caused by the years of abuse. I also saw that while alcohol harms the brain, the medication I was taking for my anxiety helped to improve my mental processing. I thanked God for the medication that helped my brain have the balance it needed after trauma so that I could move forward and learn to trust Him.

With the counseling and medicine combined, I thought I was doing all I needed to do to keep moving from victim to survivor.

But I needed to be educated more directly about what anxiety is (naming it as an "it"). I needed to understand the staggering toll it was taking on my body and why strategies to control it were so important, before it completely destroyed me.

SEEING TRUTH CLEARLY

Imagine how excited I was when my Christian counselor told me that relinquishing my anxiety to God is *giving God my state of mind*. Though my world will still cause me anxiety, I can keep giving all my worry and anxiety to God.

And regarding my identity? I am a follower of Jesus. I am a child of God. Therefore, the growth and transformation that the Holy Spirit undertakes in my life won't end until I go to be with Him.

In order to maintain all the progress I had made in recovery, and in order to move forward in my recovery, I had to do two things. First, I had to recognize and understand what this anxiety was within me. And second, I had to acknowledge that I needed better tools to fight it.

As I look back now, I see my anxiety as an effort to hide my shame. I felt ashamed of allowing someone to do such horrible things to me, for so long, without stopping it, without holding my abuser accountable. I see now that I had fallen into a deep pit of shame, thinking that because I had "failed" in these ways, I was a bad person and needed to keep trying to be better, trying, trying, trying to be perfect. It never worked.

Again, it was a matter of identity. When I saw that I was a child of God who had lived through traumatic experiences, I was better able to give my anxiety to Him.

Finally, I saw this all as a spiritual battle and began turning to God for help. With His strength I fought against the thoughts the enemy wanted to bring into my mind. I saw that part of my confusion came from the stronghold my abuser still had in my mind.

Back when I was trying to put these pieces together on my own, what the enemy wanted to convince me of seemed reasonable. The more I thought about verses such as Philippians 4:6, the more I questioned what God was asking me to do. But now I know Satan wanted to confuse me on the relevance of this Bible verse.

I've come to understand that instead of simply telling a clinically diagnosed anxious person "Don't be anxious," we can help them understand that God uses our adversity and trials to help us grow in our faith. We can tell them that a life free of anxiety can be our goal as we learn to trust Him more. God expects us to obey His Word and trust Him. He doesn't expect our "walk in the Spirit" to be flawless at all times, but He expects us to be continually growing and progressing. God didn't expect me to all of a sudden not be anxious; He expected me to learn to trust Him more and more and turn my situations over to Him. This process would decrease my anxiety.

Knowing that God loves me and wants me, anxiety and all, allowed me to feel so much closer to Him with so much more freedom in my identity in Him.

I find it so comforting to know that God doesn't expect me to be perfect in all that I do; He wants me to love Him and draw near to Him and experience His love for me. He wants me to walk in the Spirit and seek His guidance in all things. If in the midst of that I still struggle with anxiety, He understands and can give me strength to endure.

CHAPTER 22

No Feelings Today

"So how are you feeling today?"

It was a familiar question from my counselor. And the answer was always the same, a slight shrug, a slight smile, and a slight shake of the head.

By this time, she knew how to interpret it.

"No feelings?"

I shook my head again.

"Okay, well, tell me about your week."

That was safer territory. As I told her about the challenges I had faced in the preceding days, she reminded me of strategies for dealing with difficult people and situations.

Safe territory.

"Would you like to talk about any of your past today? You know, start peeling back the layers of that onion? Any thoughts? Any emotions?"

"No, not really," I replied, holding my arms tight up against my body. "I can't remember most of it, you know."

"Well, it's still in there somewhere," she observed.

Slight shrug. Slight smile.

That was territory I wasn't going to touch. It was way too painful. And besides, I really didn't remember much of it. Wasn't it better to keep it locked up in a box in the far recesses of my mind?

If my counselors would just repeat their recommended coping strategies over and over, if they would just repeat how to implement them over and over, my brain's struggles with short-term memory problems would improve.

If they would just give me very clear reasons for the coping strategies they presented, reasons that would motivate me to implement them, it would be good enough.

I reminded myself of these thoughts every time I left a counseling session.

THE LIE: I DON'T NEED TO EXPLORE MY EMOTIONS

Over the past ten years, I've met off and on with five different counselors. These professionals, with their information and resources, have helped me break down a lot of the confusion in my head. They have freed me from many of the chains of abuse that continued to hold me captive. I could now see the truth of the abuse and its results. I learned coping strategies. And with the help of the Christian counselor, I better understand the Christian faith.

Every time I succeeded in implementing a new strategy for my recovery, such as learning boundaries or how to deal with triggers, I felt a great sense of accomplishment.

So why didn't I feel fully healed?

Was I asking for too much?

Why, after all that deliberate effort toward recovery, why did I still feel like an outsider trying to live in this world? Why didn't I get spontaneous laughter and love of life back?

Should I have just been happy with the advances I'd made and the better life I'd found?

A GLIMMER OF TRUTH

When I was living in the abuse, I had learned to agree with my abuser to keep the peace. Bit by bit I had begun to believe the terrible claims he made about me—it had been easier to believe that I was to blame for everything than to acknowledge that he could be such a monstrously cruel person.

I didn't know it, but I now realize I had become brainwashed.

I didn't know it, but even after years of learning coping mechanisms, most of my thoughts, especially the subconscious ones, still functioned as if I was living in the abusive environment.

The fact of the matter was, for the first several years of my recovery, all I could focus on was whatever was happening right at the time, keeping myself and my children safe from all the potentially unsafe situations around us. And in the meantime, my body held the pain of the horrors of my experiences locked tightly in a deep, dark, inaccessible place.

If it wasn't for God's loving prodding to keep me moving forward, there's a good chance I might have accepted "feeling better" and talked myself out of setting higher goals, aiming for greater healing.

But my quiet time with God kept reminding me that He didn't die to provide an okay life for me. He died to empower me through His Holy Spirit to fulfill the destiny He has called me to.

After prayer and deep reflection, I started working on identifying why my mind believed one thing while my body was indicating another.

SEEING TRUTH CLEARLY

As it turns out, no one (that I recall) had ever told me that my inability to remember the abuse or feel any emotions indicated something significant. I later learned that my mind had disconnected from the pain because it was too hard for me to bear—a normal response for trauma survivors.

I had to bring forward and remember some extremely painful memories. I had to acknowledge that when my abuser left, he didn't take these traumatic memories with him. They just got pushed aside because remembering them was too painful.

And that situation was not sustainable for my body and my health.

If I had been listening to someone else's story instead of living my own, I would never have guessed how difficult it could be to acknowledge that my first marriage wasn't emotionally or physically healthy. In fact, acknowledging those words to a therapist devastated me, sending me into a weeks-long depression.

But eventually I had to recognize the deep effects of trauma in my life. There was no other way to move forward.

SPEAKING TRUTH:
THE UGLINESS OF TRAUMA

MYSTERIOUS SYMPTOMS

The ninth year into my recovery effort, two years after my nervous breakdown, I hit a significant roadblock. The more I tried to integrate myself into my family and environment, the more I realized how my view of the world was impacting my ability to live. After years of trying new things, venturing outside my comfort zone, expanding my boundaries, and willingly engaging in social conversations, my health took a massive decline, with sudden, mysterious, and alarming symptoms.

During my morning prayer and Bible time, my physical ailments kept reminding me that there was something I needed to pay attention to. Here I was trying to figure out how to interact better in my world, and God kept circling me around to my new physical issues.

Thank goodness God pushed me through to the next pieces of my recovery. Here I was, so close to unlocking another door to my freedom, and I almost settled for okay. God sent me on another journey to find out why my body was screaming for attention.

COPING STRATEGIES IS ONLY PART OF THE PACKAGE

What I didn't realize until I tried to integrate myself back into society despite feeling withdrawn and uninterested, is that learning coping strategies for dealing with my current world (empowerment, boundaries, triggers, and so on) is only part of the road to recovery.

The other part involves dealing with the horrors of the past held in a subconscious portion of my brain. Reading *The Body Keeps the Score: Brain, Mind, and Body in the Healing of Trauma,* by Dr. Bessel van der Kolk, provided me with much clarity and understanding of how my body had stored the trauma from twenty-one years of abuse.

HOW THE BODY IS AFFECTED BY TRAUMA

The Body Keeps the Score explains that the traumatic stress from years of abuse is deeply hidden in my body. The fact that I didn't remember the abuse and had no emotions about it indicated my brain's trauma response: a basic drive for survival had put my brain on autopilot to allow me to continue to function.

But the trauma was killing me slowly. Receiving no break from anxiety caused stress hormones to be released throughout my body for years. Without any conscious awareness on my part, this hidden traumatic stress was destroying my physical body.

HOW THE EMOTIONS ARE AFFECTED

People with whom I shared my journey would often comment on how strong I was. But I didn't feel strong. I felt numb. I felt shut down. I felt like I was existing but not enjoying the great life God offered me.

I looked but didn't see.

I listened but didn't hear.

I touched but didn't feel.

I ate but didn't taste.

Is this the way other people interact with their world? I wondered.

Years of living in such a heightened state of fear, the book explains, caused my brain to rewire. This means that even though my body was experiencing life in the current realm, I processed most of my thoughts as if I were responding to my previously abusive world.

Imagine the internal struggle I felt as my body tried to function in the present while my mind responded from my abused past. This was my struggle for so many years, causing me to feel withdrawn and like an outsider, watching the world unfold around me.

PART FOUR

FINAL LIES BLOCKING A LIFE OF PEACE

SPEAKING TRUTH: THE IMPORTANCE OF TRAUMA THERAPY

FRUSTRATIONS WITH THE LIMITATIONS OF PTSD

Knowing that I have PTSD and realizing the implications it has on my world are two entirely different pains.

Up until this point in my recovery, I had tried to ignore my PTSD. I learned how to work around it, but not how to recognize it for what it represents: I was traumatized to the point that the way I thought and interacted with my surroundings was significantly altered.

Here I was, years into recovery, so close to being able to enjoy my environment again, finally able to see what I wanted, yet so frustrated with the limitations caused by PTSD. I didn't know how to bridge that gap.

I didn't work this hard just to be "okay," content to live within the confines of my PTSD. For me, being "okay" implied I submitted to my abuser and settled for less because of him. If I didn't push the limits to find out what I could accomplish, I would have felt like a mountain climber who had stopped halfway up.

I was angry.

And besides, why hadn't my weekly counseling sessions with the traditional behavior modification therapy worked to remove the trauma from my body?

It was time for a treatment program that specialized in trauma.

TRAUMA TREATMENT PROGRAMS

Many different trauma treatment programs have proliferated in recent decades, such as EMDR (Eye Movement Desensitization and Reprocessing), Cognitive Processing Therapy, Intensive Trauma Therapy, Transformation Prayer Ministry, and neurofeedback. Instead of simply relying on what my counselor recommended, I researched treatment options to find one that I thought would best fit my needs and recovery goals.

As I prayed, the Lord confirmed where I should go with this important piece of my recovery.

OVERVIEW OF MY TRAUMA THERAPY

The trauma treatment program I entered allowed me to open up my subconscious and remove the poisonous thoughts.

- *First,* the therapist helped me "dig up" the old memories. There was no other way to be healed from the pain. The secrets had to come out of the recesses of my mind.

- *Then* I needed to acknowledge that these memories were real and allow myself to feel them. This brought with it a lot of pain, anxiety, and emotional numbness.

- *Then* I had to call them out for what they really were. This means I finally fully acknowledged the abuse and pain.

- ⊙ *Then* the memories were reprocessed, seen with truth instead of lies. I had to relive the memories to bring forward those deeply hidden assumptions, so they could be reprocessed this time in a compassionate, healthier manner.

- ⊙ *Then* I could put them safely and slowly back into my memory bank, fully processed.

The whole experience, with one memory after another, was very difficult and painful, but not so painful that I wanted to give up. In fact, I felt motivated and validated, knowing that there was indeed so much hidden in my mind that I needed to reprocess from a healthy standpoint before it destroyed me more.

Still, the numbness, inability to function, and overall depressing feelings were surely acknowledgment of how painful my past was. My mood was so volatile during these weeks! Once I started opening the floodgate of memories, they seemed to occur randomly throughout my day.

ALLOWING BODY MEMORIES

Working through this treatment plan was extremely hard; physically, my body responded as if I were being abused again, in what are called "body memories." Fortunately, the trauma therapist warned me about how my body would react when the old thoughts were moved forward.

DISMANTLING LIES

The daily homework allowed for me to slowly pull the secrets from my past into my current thought processes, to look at each memory and call it out for what it really was: abusive.

Realizing that the experience was abusive, I could safely reprocess the thought this time with a disclaimer, like this:

- My abuser did what he did to me not because of something defective in me, but because he was an abuser.

- My abuser abused me because he wanted to exert power and control over me.

- My abuser did what he did because he wanted to, regardless of what I tried to do or not do to remedy the situation.

- After the memory had been reprocessed, it could be put back into my memory bank.

RESULTS OF THE THERAPY

CHANGING HABITUAL THOUGHT PATTERNS

Throughout my trauma therapy, I obtained a good look at how many of my thought patters were based on habits created by brainwashing, rather than facts. When I identified these habitual thoughts, I realized that my entire worldview was being challenged. I spent many weeks tearing these thoughts apart, identifying what was brainwashing and what was fact.

Reprograming my thoughts required me to:

- analyze every thought I had to see if it was true or false,

- rebut the lies associated with the way my abuser had taught me to think,

- process the thought with truth, and then

- believe the truth.

Believing the truth, repeating it over and over again until it became an automatic thought, required hours of focus and repetition. Breaking apart twenty-one years of lies about myself from my abuser took months of hard work.

Yes, it was hard work. Yes, it was exhausting. But it was worth it. Here are examples of some of the thoughts I reprocessed.

REFUSING SELF-CONDEMNING THOUGHTS

I finally was able to tear apart all those repetitive slurs that had been rattling around in the back of my mind all these years. Insults like: *you are so selfish, incompetent, can't do anything right, horrible wife and mother, overall terrible human being.*

Finally, I could take these brainwashed invectives and separate them from my current world. I could trace them to the source and refute them with truth.

ACKNOWLEDGING MY OWN STRENGTH

Over the past few years as I have started to talk about my abuse, people have looked at me and seen strength. Over and over again, I have felt weakness.

People have repeatedly commented that they thought I handled the abuse, along with our daughter's cancer, with poise. Never once did I ever credit myself with being strong; instead, I felt like I did what I needed to do to survive.

When I was in the abuse, I was never able to process the abusive events, as constant and sudden and fast-paced as they were.

Even after I was out of the abuse, I still felt like I was bouncing around doing what my abuser ordered; I never felt like I was in control of anything.

But trauma therapy allowed me to look deeply at this disconnect between what people were seeing and what I was feeling.

What if those painful diatribes from my abuser were meant to burst the strength that he saw in me even in that living nightmare?

For the first time in my life, I finally began giving myself credit for what I had endured.

NO LONGER LIVING IN CRISIS MODE

During this therapy I identified how I still mentally process events with crisis mode tendencies even though my current world was calm and safe. I thought about every "what if," turning routine events into crisis situations, increasing the level of my own stress and the stress of others around me.

Part of learning to speak the truth was reminding myself I am no longer with my abuser and I will process my circumstances based on the present rather than the past.

RENEWING TRUST

Long-term abuse had left me feeling like I couldn't trust anyone. If the man I loved, the father of my three children, could harm me in such a way that I was so deeply tormented, then how could I possibly trust anyone?

Yet during trauma therapy I realized that I can trust people, just not my abusive ex-husband. How freeing to find out that the entire world isn't untrustworthy, just my abuser!

Yes, there will be times when I'll meet someone untrustworthy, but I know I don't need to jump to the conclusion that most people are bad until they prove to be safe. I am learning to trust people first.

REINTEGRATING INTO SOCIETY

After reading John 8:12[3], I knew that continuing to live in my safe and limited world was not what God wanted for me. He wanted me to enjoy this newfound freedom and security that He had provided. He wanted me to be a witness for others to emulate, not a person who remained stuck living in her past.

At first, forcing myself out of my comfort zone to interact with others felt overwhelming. I had grown accustomed to simply observing events in my life rather than being a part of them. It was too hard to trust people, so was it really in my best interest to leave the comforts of my home to go out to do things and engage in ordinary conversation with others?

Ironically, the coping skills I had used to offset my PTSD (avoidance of crowds or new events) also constricted my ability to do things.

Opening this door in my mind took deliberate action and praying on my part. I used the tools I had learned in trauma therapy, especially dismantling the lies. This way I was able to begin making conscious decisions to encourage myself to get out and do things. To genuinely enjoy my new life, the one I had worked so hard for, I had to get out of my house and experience new environments.

I started with small situations to try to reintegrate myself back into my community, which meant I had to relearn certain social skills, such as small talk. I was surprised at how hard this was for me.

However, I knew I couldn't live in isolation—it's not good for faith accountability or personal growth. I knew it would limit my opportunities to show God's great grace. I also knew that the best way to enjoy the newfound calmness and peace in my heart was to get out and experience it in new situations. This was also the way I

---

3   John 8:12 says, "When Jesus spoke again to the people, he said, "I am the light of the world. Whoever follows me will never walk in darkness, but will have the light of life."

was going to be able to tell and show others how faithful God has been to me.

Getting out of my comfort zone has been worth it.

LIVING IN THE PRESENT TENSE

When I started this therapy, I felt withdrawn from the real world as my mind continuously remained in the past.

Trauma treatment counseling allowed me to retrain my mind and body to be able to fully live in the here and now. I even began to focus on talking positively about the present: "This is fun" versus "That was fun."

It took a lot of work, but I finally learned that it was okay to let go of my past. I don't have to constantly contemplate crisis scenarios. I don't have to condemn myself. I don't have to be afraid. I can live in—and even enjoy—the moment.

Eventually, I started smiling.

Then the day came when I heard myself laugh. My laughter is now a common occurrence, but at that time, it sounded so strange to me and caught me so off guard that I didn't even recognize it.

FACING THE GUILT AND SHAME

There's one more thing I did as I processed my trauma therapy. I made a conscious effort to address the underlying guilt that I hadn't handled things well during my marriage to Tom. I had to let go of the shame embedded in many of those memories. I had to let go of the guilt that I stayed in the relationship too long. I had to let go of all the guilt of the could haves, should haves, and would haves that were left within my mind.

Once again, I had to receive the forgiveness that God offered me through His Son, Jesus Christ. If God forgave me, then surely I could forgive myself and release the entrapment of my guilt and shame.

OTHER APPROACHES FOR DECREASING TRAUMA EFFECTS

SYNCHRONIZING MIND AND BODY

I read that one of the effects of trauma is that victims no longer feel safe within their bodies. I could relate to this, as I was physically violated so many times. I lost trust in my ability to protect myself, which was especially evident when I was in large crowds. This feeling led to the dissociation from my body I often experienced.

When I would stretch before riding an exercise bike, I would go through the motions, but my mind was still racing. I thought about how tired I was, how hungry I was, or how I needed to hurry to start exercising because I needed to go somewhere else.

Before I started learning about the benefits yoga provides to trauma survivors, it looked to me like stretching exercises. Although this is true, I now know that the primary difference between standard stretching exercises and yoga is working the body and mind together at the same time, in unison.

The impact of focusing on my breathing became plainly evident, the scattered thoughts disappeared almost immediately and my mind stopped racing.

Focusing on my movement brought me a new awareness of my body. As my body and breathing became synchronized and stronger, I could tell my body what to do, and my body obeyed.

Becoming more aware of my body also made me more conscious of my aches and pains. As a result, I began to be able to recognize some cause and effect connections when it came to my physical ailments. For example, focusing on stretching out my neck and shoulder muscles significantly decreased my headaches. As I have learned to focus on my body, I'm now able to help heal the parts of my body that have held stress.

FOCUS ON BREATHING TO CALM MYSELF

Earlier in my recovery, I realized that since my head had been injured multiple times during the abuse, I should respect it and care for it. After all, I reasoned, if my ankle had been injured, it would be standard protocol to elevate it and rest it.

So I wondered if resting my head after an anxious moment or day would be better for me than trying to fight the anxiety. I found that fifteen minutes of uninterrupted, calm, quiet resting greatly assisted in my ability to get through a situation. Come to find out, the resting of my head was a calming technique for my racing mind.

Focusing on breathing as a way to calm oneself and quiet the thoughts is sometimes called meditation. Given that I struggle daily to keep my anxiety under control, I focus on my breathing as I work around the house or drive. This greatly assists me in calming a racing thought. After I started focusing on my breathing lying in bed, I found it a lot easier to fall asleep.

Being in touch with my breathing reminds me of how thankful I am to be alive. I am breathing. I am alive.

CHAPTER 23

COFFEE CHAT WITH GOD

For the most part, my favorite time of my day is sitting in my recliner, with my dogs curled up next to me, drinking my morning coffee and chatting with God. When I first found out that someone wanted to listen to me, I was so excited. What a true friend to spend my morning coffee time with.

However, talking with God was one thing. Reading the Bible was something else entirely different. I knew from the pastor's sermons that to be a good Christian I needed to read and understand God's Word. I saw people in church carrying worn-out Bibles—they were obviously reading theirs.

But many mornings after reading my Bible, I felt confused, defeated, like less of a Christian, and ready to give up on trying to learn God's Word.

I remember reading the book of James and coming across the following:

James 1:2: *"Consider it pure joy, my brothers and sisters, whenever you face trials of many kinds...."*

This passage concerned me so much that, if I remember correctly, I stopped reading the Bible for a couple of weeks. Instead, I just drank my coffee and talked to God in the morning. I wasn't going to give that up, but it seemed so much easier to skip reading the confusing Bible verses than trying to figure out what they meant.

How could I be joyful for the pain I suffered from my abuser? I definitely wasn't going to be excited when more trials attacked me. I had no trouble telling God how I truly felt about that.

The Lie: "Some Bible commands are impossible to obey"

James 1:2 wasn't the only bible verse that seemed impossible. How about these verses?

Luke 6:27-28: *"But to you who are listening I say: Love your enemies, do good to those who hate you, bless those who curse you, pray for those who mistreat you."*[4]

How was I supposed to do that while keeping my boundaries in place?

Or what about these?

Romans 12:17-18: *"Do not repay anyone evil for evil. Be careful to do what is right in the eyes of everyone. If it is possible, as far as it depends on you, live at peace with everyone."*[5]

How could I do that when my abuser continued to take advantage of every situation to topple me?

The more I asked for God's help, the more I became confused about my faith. How was it possible that a God who tells me to love my enemy, be a peacemaker, and be anxious for nothing was possibly going to understand my predicament?

Yes, I would follow God, but there was no way possible I could honor such hard commands. Obviously, God didn't know the hellish conditions I had been living in. Or if He did, he evidently didn't care enough to stop the abuse.

---

4   Discussed in Chapter 24.
5   Discussed in Chapter 25.

It was not remotely possible that I should be required to do such things.

And forgiveness? Now God had me confused with someone who hadn't lived through such horrors.

I felt defeated again. The devil was doing everything possible to hinder my spiritual growth. Sometimes it felt easier to give up and let the devil and the emotional abuse win.

WHERE WAS THE CHURCH?

By now I'd been reading the Bible and going to church for years. I thought for sure reading the Bible and finding a healthy church would be the answer to my prayers for recovering from my domestic violence past.

I must admit, though, as helpful as church was, often I left a church service in more pain than when I arrived. For some reason, I found many sermons superficial, confusing, and not digging into the deep issues that haunted me. It seemed that the church message I was hearing didn't address issues from my perspective as a victim. Yes, the Sunday sermons told me what I should be doing, but I didn't hear the how-to steps. What was it that God really wanted me to do, given my victim perspective on the world?

As I turned to the church for assistance, I immediately felt defeated again. As I diligently searched for support in the form of a Bible study, I found nothing. In my medium-sized southern city it seemed there were countless Bible studies going on; yet I couldn't find a Bible study for domestic violence victims. How could this be possible when statistics reveal that one out of every four females in the United States will be subjected to severe physical abuse?

I felt rejected again.

My feeling of rejection stung harshly. The reality that the Church wasn't interested enough in my recovery to at least put together a Bible study for domestic violence victims was extremely distressing.

I looked for Christian literature to help me with my confusion. Once again, I couldn't find anything that explained—from a Christian perspective—how to transition from victim to survivor.

In the absence of church support, my faith was becoming unbearably confusing. The overall lack of support I perceived deflated my persistence to find answers to my complicated questions. I almost gave up my search for the real answers to my confusion.

A GLIMMER OF TRUTH

Fortunately God's desire to grow in my heart wouldn't allow me to be defeated. In the absence of the resources I so desperately sought, God gave me the strength and relentless determination to persevere until I found the answers to the questions He had so strategically placed in my heart.

The voice in my heart provided me with two options: remain angry and confused (in which Satan wins) or continue to seek out what God was guiding me to do.

I decided not to give up on my search for answers.

After many mornings of prayer, I started to realize that part of the reason I was having a hard time understanding the Bible was because the emotional and spiritual abuse I had endured continued to interject negative thoughts into my mind.

I also knew my beginner's understanding of the Bible was flawed due to the continuing influence of the emotional abuse, so I solicited God's assistance even more. His continuous influence in my life brought me to the point of questioning my interpretation of these verses.

Quiet times during my devotion pushed me further: what if I actually misunderstood some verses that were essential to my recovery? What if the tainted view I had of my world was manipulating my ability to understand what the Bible was telling me to do?

One day, in God's providence, I bumped into my church's associate pastor at the store, and he asked why he hadn't seen me in a while. I took that opportunity to follow up with a meeting with him.

Turned out I was right—there was no church support for domestic violence survivors. But this associate pastor guided me to a Christian counselor who ended up being a lifesaver to me.

Over the ten months that I met with this counselor (before she had to move out of state), we broke down the Scriptures in the next chapters.

Because of these counseling sessions, the enemy's strongholds in my mind began to shatter more. My faith became clearer and stronger.

CHAPTER 24

ON THE PHONE AT THE BASEBALL GAME

By the time my younger son was a junior in high school, the man who had abused me for so many years was experiencing declining health. It had been two years since Tom had stopped driving. His ability to get out of his house and do ordinary activities was becoming extremely difficult.

I would arrive at my son's baseball games excited to watch him play. I admit I was also excited to be able to watch the game without my abuser around.

It's hard to say what my motivation really was, but when my abuser called throughout my son's baseball games I believed the Christian thing to do was to answer the phone. It was not unusual for Tom to call me three or four times throughout the game, in addition to once more for a recap at the end. When our son did something noteworthy on the field, I even sometimes found myself calling Tom to tell him.

It seemed like the Christian thing to do. But by the time I left the field, I felt strung out, with my thoughts rattling. Eventually, I became conflicted. Was I talking to Tom on the phone because I thought it was the right thing to do (loving my enemy) or was it because I was afraid if I didn't talk to him he would get mad?

That part didn't matter; he got mad anyway.

But then, how was I supposed to obey Scriptures like these?

Luke 6:27-28: *"But to you who are listening I say: Love your enemies, do good to those who hate you, bless those who curse you, pray for those who mistreat you."*

THE LIE: I CAN'T LOVE MY ENEMY

The hardest biblical verse for me to understand and accept was the concept of loving my enemy. In the early stages of my newfound faith, I thought for sure this command was meant for other people, not for those of us whose boundaries had been so violently violated. How could it be remotely possible that God is instructing me to love someone who hurt me so badly? I used to love my abuser, and look where that got me: physically, emotionally, and sexually abused.

When I thought of the word *love*, I related it to my current husband, my mom, my children, and those close to me. I saw love as a mutual, positive, give-and-take relationship. I saw it as involving two sides that were mutually respectful and working toward keeping the relationship alive and fulfilling.

Although I loved my current husband differently than I loved my children, I still saw love as an emotional response to important people in my life. How was it possible to share that emotion with my abuser? How could I possibly love my enemy?

Another problem I was having in loving my enemy was that I thought the many ways I used the word *love* (I love brownies, I love my husband and my children, I love my job) all conveyed basically the same meaning, having to do with the love "bringing me plea-sure." Even though I knew, of course, that things like brownies and jobs can't reciprocate the feelings to have an actual relationship, I still thought that the intensity of the feeling of love was directly tied to the amount of pleasure the thing or person provided to me. The greater the pleasure, the greater the love.

So with that line of thinking, how was it possible to love my enemy? How was it possible to love someone who was not going to show any appreciation or affection back, who was not going to give me the least little bit of pleasure?

The only other idea I could come up with—since that one didn't work—was that I was supposed to put his needs before mine, no matter how much he hurt me. This was the way, I figured (and the negative voices in my head confirmed), to love my enemy.

But it didn't work; it never worked. All my abuser wanted was to manipulate my thoughts and actions; his "needs" were devilish. All my efforts to show love by putting his needs before mine backfired.

I thought that just in general, being a Christian meant I put other people's needs before mine. How could I possibly put my abuser's needs before mine?

I thought being a Christian meant I should do whatever it took to help someone out. You know what happened when I tried to apply these principles toward my abuser? He immediately turned the situation/conversation into an argument and often an attack. When I tried to open the door to help him, the only thing I got was more anxiety and confusion.

What did I get in return for being nice, pleasant, and accommodating? Nothing positive. What did I get for being a team player who did everything I could to show my children how to communicate positively with their dad? Nothing but anxiety and emotional turmoil.

I was trying everything I knew to do right...without grasping the correct meaning of these verses from the Bible.

I sank into pain and confusion, believing that this Bible command was impossible to obey.

Eventually, I settled for doing my best to be non-confrontational toward my abuser. This was the most I could accomplish.

A GLIMMER OF TRUTH

The light dawned for me when I learned the true meanings for our English word *love* from my Christian counselor. The Greek language used in the Bible has four different words for the four different kinds of love God describes in His Word.

The ancient Greeks had four words for different types of love.

Phileo is the affectionate feeling we have towards our friends and people close to us. "This love speaks of affection, fondness, and liking."[6]

Storge is family love. *Storge* is the love I have toward my mom, my sisters, and my children. "It is a quiet, abiding feeling within a [person] that rests on something close to him and that he feels good about."[7]

Eros is erotic love, "bedroom" love. *Eros* is "a love that is an emotional involvement based on body chemistry."[8]

Agape is Christ-like love. "This love keeps on loving even when the loved one is unresponsive, unkind, unlovable and unworthy. It is unconditional love." There are very few instances of this word for love outside the Bible, but in the Bible, it's used often. *Agape* is the love God wants all His children to show others because everyone is made in the image of God.[9]

---

6   Kenneth S. Wuest. *Wuest's Word Studies in the Greek New Testament, Vol. III* (Grand Rapids, MI: William B. Eerdmans Publishing Co.,1984), 111-113.

7   Ibid.

8   Ibid.

9   Ibid.

SEEING TRUTH CLEARLY

This is why I was having such a hard time with loving my enemy: I thought I was supposed to love my enemy with the same type of love I was demonstrating toward my current husband and my children. But I learned that this is not the kind of love God is asking me to share with my abuser. God is not asking me to express the emotional component of love toward my abuser as I do when I express *phileo*, *storge*, or *eros*.

He is asking me to show *agape*, compassion, the kind of love we are called to show toward all people.

WHAT DOES LOVE WITH BOUNDARIES LOOK LIKE?

1 Peter 4:8-9 says, *"Above all, love [agape] each other deeply, because love covers over a multiple of sins. Offer hospitality to one another without grumbling."*

This Scripture was clarified for me by Proverbs 25:21: *"If your enemy is hungry, give him food to eat; if he is thirsty, give him water to drink."*

This verse provided me with the parameters that I needed in order to understand how I was supposed to love and interact with my abuser. Understanding this kind of love means that I will do what I can to ensure that any person God puts in my path has food and water, a roof over their head, and access to medical treatment if possible.

Putting this verse into perspective did much to quiet the noise in my head.

When I do show this kind of love (even if I continue to keep myself safe while I do it), I am then demonstrating that I respect my abuser as a person and want to see that he is treated with dignity, as every person should be. I acknowledge and even appreciate the fact that God made him and loves him.

It does *not* mean that all is forgotten or that I will expose myself to being hurt again.

LIVING FOR GOD RATHER THAN MAN

Because Christian love is an act of will, it involves maturity in my faith and my actions. It involves following God's guidance, even if it means taking the hard right over the easy wrong.

When I use an act of will to love my abuser in the way God has called me to love him, treating him with respect as one created in God's image, then I can do it without any expectations from my abuser. I focus on God and what God has asked me to do and refuse to open myself up to Tom's ridicule. Approaching situations with my abuser this way allows me to focus on the task at hand and as soon as that task is over, I move on and away from my abuser.

CHAPTER 25

I CAN'T DO WHAT GOD IS ASKING ME TO DO

When it came to medical decisions for our children, I could never do anything right.

I could never. Do anything. Right.

"Honestly," I prayed through gritted teeth, "can't the kids just keep quiet about their ailments when they have visitation with him? I can handle it all as long as I don't have to answer to their dad for it."

So now I stood in a specialty clinic with my son, who suffered from mysterious nausea (which was later diagnosed as Crohn's disease). Of course, according to my abuser, I wasn't getting him through the specialty clinics fast enough.

Just like when my oldest child's appendix burst, it was all my fault because I took him to the emergency room too late.

Just like when my daughter's permanent teeth were blocked from coming in by the baby teeth that refused to fall out (residual effects of childhood radiation), it was, of course, due to my slowness in taking her to the dentist.

So I stood there looking at the "authorized contacts" blanks, fuming. My ex-husband never did anything to help with the medical needs. He only blamed and accused.

On impulse, instead of writing in the father's name, I wrote in the name of the children's stepfather.

Ha! I thought. That will show him. But I didn't think he would actually find out.

I was wrong. Somehow he did discover what I had done, and as would be expected, I received another horrible verbal assault.

After so many years of being hurt, it felt so much easier—and more empowering—to hurt him even in small ways than to forgive him of all the hurt and pain he had caused me.

THE LIE: I CAN'T REALLY FORGIVE SOMEONE WHO CAUSED ME SO MUCH PAIN

I was gaining a new sense of strength and self-confidence. I was learning how to influence aspects of my environment, through my understanding of triggers and boundaries, to control and lessen my pain. I was setting controls on things I had once thought were uncontrollable.

And it felt good. I felt alive. I felt alive for the first time in twenty-five years.

So in my mind it only made sense that if I was feeling stronger, I should use that strength against the one who had abused me for so long. I began to think I should be holding my abuser responsible for all the years of abuse he put me through.

I was pretty sure my abuser wasn't agonizing every day about the harm he caused me; he wasn't concerned about how my life had been turned upside down.He would continue to do anything to make my life miserable. He didn't have morals or boundaries so he didn't care what he did as long as it would negatively impact my world. He would degrade me whenever the situation arose, whenever he felt like it.

I knew the Bible talked about forgiveness, like this verse:

Colossians 3:13: *"Bear with each other and forgive one another if any of you has a grievance against someone. Forgive as the Lord forgave you."*

When my children were young and misbehaved, it never occurred to me to stop, breathe, forgive, and then handle the situation.

No, I would punish them first, and then forgive their bad behavior. Often the forgiveness was even contingent on their response to the punishment. The longer my kids moped and complained, the longer it took me to forgive the situation and move on. This is the same way I felt about my abuser.

I knew forgiving was important. But that was the only way I knew how to "forgive."

A GLIMMER OF TRUTH

Because I was regularly reading the Bible, I kept on being stopped by difficult verses, verses that didn't make sense in my world.

Matthew 6:14-15 states: *"For if you forgive other people when they sin against you, your heavenly Father will also forgive you. But if you do not forgive others their sins, your Father will not forgive your sins."*

During the early years of my recovery, this was a hard and confusing sermon for me to listen to in church, from a hard and confusing passage of Scripture. My abuser's crimes were so atrocious I believed I could never fully forgive them the way God was asking.

The parable of the unmerciful servant in Matthew 18 helped clarify what God was asking me to do.

Matthew 18:21: *"Peter came to Jesus and asked, 'Lord, how many times shall I forgive my brother or sister who sins against me? Up to seven times?'"*

Peter wanted to keep track of how many times he was being sinned against. At the time, the rabbis taught that it was appropriate to forgive three times, so offering forgiveness an additional four times may have made Peter feel more faithful. Jesus answered.

Matthew 18:22: *"Jesus answered, "I tell you, not seven times, but seventy-seven times."*

If I had been told this, I would probably be caught off guard. Imagine having to forgive my abuser so many times! Surely this seems excessive. But that was Jesus' point. If we learn to forgive someone this many times, we have probably mastered the art of forgiveness the way God intended us to live.

The parable goes on to illustrate this act of forgiveness in Matthew 18:23-35:

Therefore, the kingdom of heaven is like a king who wanted to settle accounts with his servants. As he began the settlement, a man who owed him ten thousand bags of gold was brought to him. Since he was not able to pay, the master ordered that he and his wife and his children and all that he had to be sold to repay the debt.

At this, the servant fell on his knees before him. "Be patient with me," he begged, "and I will pay back everything." The servant's master took pity on him, canceled the debt and let him go.

But when that servant went out, he found one of his fellow servants who owed him a hundred silver coins. He grabbed him and began to choke him. "Pay back what you owe me!" he demanded.

His fellow servant fell to his knees and begged him, "Be patient with me, and I will pay it back."

But he refused. Instead, he went off and had the man thrown into prison until he could pay the debt. When the other servants saw what had happened, they were outraged and went and told their master everything that had happened.

Then the master called the servant in. "You wicked servant," he said, "I canceled that debt of yours because you begged me to. Shouldn't you have had mercy on your fellow servant just as I had on you?" In anger his master handed him over to the jailers to be tortured, until he should pay back all he owed.

This is how my heavenly Father will treat each of you unless you forgive your brother or sister from your heart.

I saw those last three words—we are to forgive from our hearts. Forgiving someone with words is easy to do. But just because the words "I forgive you" came out of my mouth didn't mean I'd forgiven anyone. The words alone didn't count for forgiveness.

Forgiving someone from the heart is the harder but more complete and real path that God was asking me to take.

SEEING TRUTH CLEARLY

LETTING GO OF DESIRES FOR REVENGE

One morning during my devotion time, God countered my misconceptions and Satan's lies with Romans 12:17-19.

"Do not repay anyone evil for evil. Be careful to do what is right in the eyes of everyone. [For me, this means doing

183

*what is right in the eyes of my children, living by example,
not just by words.] If it is possible, as far as it depends on
you, live at peace with everyone. Do not take revenge,
my dear friends, but leave room for God's wrath, for it is
written: 'It is mine to avenge; I will repay?' says the Lord."*

My world stopped for a minute. Was it remotely possible that
God would fight my abuser for me? Really? No one had ever held my
abuser accountable for what he had done.

That verse stopped me in my tracks. In the absence of using the
judicial system, it looked like someone was going to hold my abuser
accountable.

I learned from Romans 12:19 that God was offering me protection: He was offering to stand up for me and fight the battles for
me in the case of someone who had harmed me and was not being
held accountable. My part was to keep my boundaries and ask for
His help.

Stepping back from the fight and learning to trust God about my
abuser's accountability was hard, and it continues to be hard. There's
no denying I sometimes wanted to go into attack mode against my
abuser, especially once I found out God would lead the charge!

But instead of responding suddenly out of my emotions when I
interacted with my abuser, I had to learn to wait for guidance in my
heart from the Lord. This has meant a total change of my mindset.
As a situation was developing, I had to listen, breathe, pray hard, and
sometimes even fast.

God's strength came internally, so that I could respond to my
abuser from a position of dignity. Quietly, calmly, and poised.

BECOMING READY FOR REAL "FORGIVENESS"

Being willing to let God exact vengeance was one thing. Being
willing to forgive was something else altogether.

So what does "forgiveness" really mean? What does God mean when He tells me to forgive?

In simple terms, it means to let go. For my forgiveness to be sincere, it needed to be a decision from my heart to let go. Total, 100 percent of the time (not just when it was convenient) letting go.

This decision to forgive my abuser was costly and difficult. I found out as it took months of hard, concentrated prayer asking for God's help to remove the pain from my heart and replace it with God's grace and peace.

I found out too that forgiveness is not a feeling; it is a decision of the will, a decision I made despite feelings of resentment or hurt. The Holy Spirit that dwells inside me provided me with the willpower to do what was right. There was no way I could forgive on my own; for me to forgive, I had to turn my thoughts and emotions to Jesus Christ and be willing by God's grace to make the decision to let go.

WHAT FORGIVENESS DOESN'T MEAN

I learned that forgiveness is not given in relationship to retaliation, wins, or hardships incurred by my enemy. Forgiveness is not something I give today, only to let the desire for revenge get in the way tomorrow. Furthermore…

Forgiveness doesn't mean I'll forget the wrongs that were done to me, nor do I need to pretend nothing happened. I will always have the memories of abuse; they are now part of my story.

Forgiveness doesn't mean I can't speak the truth about what my abuser did to me. But it means I'll speak the truth with grace, refusing to couple these words with words of revenge or unrighteous anger.

Forgiveness doesn't mean I'll trust my abuser again. If someone wrecked your car out of negligence, you could forgive them for that wreck, but that doesn't necessarily mean you would allow them to borrow your car again.

Forgiveness doesn't mean I'll make myself vulnerable to my abuser again. God has asked me to remove myself from evildoers, not to continue to be manipulated by them. If you told something confidential about yourself to a coworker and then found that coworker had spread it all over the office, you can forgive that coworker without ever again communicating personal information to him or her.

Forgiveness doesn't mean I need to have a relationship with the person I'm forgiving. No words are even required to forgive; I didn't need to say anything to my abuser to forgive him. I could forgive Tom from my heart without ever telling him "I forgive you."

WHEN THE TIME IS RIGHT

Though forgiving was an essential step in my journey, it wasn't one I could have accomplished at some predetermined time in my recovery. Well-meaning Christians, knowing that forgiveness is one of the most important parts of the journey to becoming a survivor, urged me early on to forgive. But trying to forgive too early, *before I even fully understood what it was I was forgiving*, would have been counterproductive.

In following the lead of the Holy Spirit, I knew when the time for forgiveness had arrived for me.

TAKING THE HARDEST STEP

The longer I held on to not forgiving, the longer my thoughts, words, and actions continued to be painfully impacted by my abuser. There came a point when I could sense it was time to embrace the potentially hardest—but for me the most rewarding—step of the recovery process, perhaps the biggest step in leaving behind the bondage of my past.

With God stirring in my heart, I began a massive campaign to truly forgive my abuser. With His help, I was able to break free from an extraordinary bondage from my past.

With forgiveness, I made the choice to release myself from the pain my abuser inflicted on me, allowing me to get on with my life instead of being trapped by resentment. Forgiveness meant I was letting go of anger, pain, resentment, malice, and vindictive thoughts and actions, and replacing them with God's truth and beauty. Surrendering all my fighting to God brought a new sense of calmness. God directed me to "let go" of the situation so He could replace my feelings of abandonment with His love and peace.

UNEXPECTED RESULTS

A NEW CALM

The strangest thing happened when I forgave my abuser. I wanted to move forward in the confidence that God's truth meant more to me than my feelings. But to my surprise, there was an added benefit: *Nothing my abuser did agitated me anymore.*

My determination to "let go" was a deliberate, hard fight that required many months, but in the end, it has been so worth it. Replacing resentment and anger with a continued determination to "let go" discharged those negative emotions that arose up at the sound of my abuser's name. Instead, I was able to focus on God's Word with a calm disposition.

I made a choice to refuse to let my abuser keep hurting me anymore. He stopped winning because I ceased to allow his words and actions to bother me. Forgiveness, the real, change-of-heart kind of forgiveness, is what finally set me free from my abuser's stronghold. It finally quieted the last bits of my abuser's commotion in my head.

FORGIVING OTHERS

The biggest impact of learning to forgive was, of course, my interactions with my abuser. But I also had to forgive a lot of other people. Most of the people I had to forgive didn't even realize that their words and actions had hurt me.

Often when someone talked to me not realizing the pain and fear I was hiding behind, I became easily offended and even angry. After the conversation or situation ended, the other person went on with their life not even realizing that I was offended, in emotional turmoil, and rehashing the situation in my mind for days or weeks. During those double-life days I interpreted their loving thoughts and ideas as criticism about my personal failure.

Once I chose to forgive people who hurt me inadvertently during those dark years, God met me, and His love took the pain of my wounds and healed them. The more I focused on forgiving, the more God's love healed me.

THE IMPACT ON MY CHILDREN

When it came to visitation, my children fared far better seeing me as a woman at peace instead of a woman needing revenge.

Now my children could see, when their dad failed them again and again, that I was there simply to support them.

Instead of interpreting their dad's actions through my complaints, when I stepped out of the way they were able to see their dad as he truly was.

When all those years of my covering for him stopped, they felt the full weight of disappointment at all his failures: when he was late, when he canceled, and when he didn't follow through on his promises.

They didn't need me to magnify their disappointments and pain at his callousness; they needed me to be there for them, someone they could talk to, someone they could trust, someone they could safely bring their disappointment and confusion to.

Yes, it was extremely difficult at times to bite my tongue, to keep from voicing my real opinion about the way my abuser was hurting his children. Besides letting my children see for themselves rather than through my "filter," I also wanted to teach them that all people should be treated with dignity and respect, even those who do not treat others that way.

I gained so much more out of simply being there for them during their confusion than I ever would have by criticizing their dad to them.

If I had harshly criticized my abuser in front of my children, should I then have been surprised if they became snappy and disrespectful to me? After all, teaching my children patience, love, and self-control starts at home. That means I needed to demonstrate those things myself, even if one child begins, for instance, to pick up the vocabulary and mocking tone of his dad. With the proper example, I've seen these kinds of things become less and less of a problem.

It also means keeping the children out of the middle of divorce, custody, visitation, and child-support battles as much as possible.

Leading by example is what Jesus did while He was here on earth. The book of John is filled with example after example of Jesus showing God's strength and love to those who believed, those who were curious, and those who were nonbelievers. Jesus' calmness, trust in His Father, and non-confrontational demeanor toward the ignorant who didn't know Him is the example for us.

GOD'S HEALING

I can't change the situations of my past. But I can change how I grow from those situations and how I use them to help me become a better Christian, wife, mother, and daughter.

For me, being a peacemaker brought a small measure of positive affirmation to my disruptive situation. Accepting my journey and forgiving my abuser released some of the enemy's final strongholds on me.

When you're ready, I hope the power of forgiveness releases you as completely as it released me.

CHAPTER 26

YOUNG MAN IN THE NURSING HOME

"Hi, Mom," I said into the phone. "How are you doing today?"

My heart felt wistful, talking to my mom five hours away, knowing she was in the nursing home, declining with Parkinson's disease. She spoke with a little confusion about what she had eaten for supper.

But I knew our nightly game would cheer her up and help her focus.

"Mom," I said, "how has God shown His love for you today?"

It never failed to brighten her. Some days it was the bird on the window ledge. Once it was the children's chorus who came and sang for them.

But tonight, tonight it was different.

"Oh, Sue, a young man came in here this afternoon," she began. "He came to help me with that doggone leg brace, but you know what else he did?"

"No, what did he do, Mom?" I loved hearing the lilt in her voice as she spoke.

"He stayed and visited with me. A long time, it seemed like... *Andy Griffith* had just ended when he got here, and he stayed until they came to get me for supper."

That meant he had come at 4:30 p.m. and stayed until 6 o'clock. He had stayed with her for an hour and a half.

"He told me stories of his family," my mom continued, laughing. "He has children, and he showed me pictures of them on his phone— I'll never get used to that, you know!—and they are the cutest little things. One of them is three and the other one is five, and he had so many funny stories. You know how cute little children are, well…"

I listened as Mom went on to tell me stories of this stranger's children. This stranger who sat with my mother for an hour and a half, even when he had family of his own to go home to, showing love and care for a lonely old woman.

THE LIE: GROWING IN FAITH IS TOO HARD

I had been thinking that growing in faith needed to be done according to a rigid step-by-step guide. Trying to do it had become stressful for me, and even, if I admit it, exhausting. At times I felt ignorant. It sometimes seemed like a tense and nerve-racking challenge with a gold-star mentality. That is, in the ongoing battle for who had control of my thoughts (myself, my abuser, or God), I could feel triumph if I succeeded (gold star) or failure if I didn't.

Like a young child learning to walk, I had fallen down a lot, but I learned how to take the bruises, adjust my strategy, and try again. Some days I did well. Some days I fumbled a lot. I tried to remain focused on the enormous effort it was going to take to retrain my thought processes to get the lies out of my head, focus on the good, and recognize all that God was doing in my life.

A GLIMMER OF TRUTH

For me, the story of the young man in the nursing home was a lesson I needed to hear. It encouraged me that my growing faith in

God could be cultivated in simple, quiet ways, by the people He puts in my life.

I knew that isolation doesn't help faith to grow. True Christian people didn't criticize me (my fear was that they would consider me stupid, the way my abuser did); instead, they welcomed me and my ignorance with open arms. True Christian people thrive on walking with new Christians to answer questions, show love, and demonstrate how to grow closer with God.

Over time, I learned that my growing faith is something that cultivates in my heart as I trust God more, lean on Him more, and look to Him in my heart.

I kept working on following God one step at a time. I had the medicine needed to calm my head, and my world was relatively safe. As I continued to grasp the importance of trusting God in my recovery, I focused more attention on where my faith in God was leading me. As I sought answers, I heard a motivating sermon one Sunday morning.

During this one particular sermon that I so vividly remember years later, our pastor broke down the foundational principles of my faith so simply. Breaking down the internalized, overwhelming size of my faith journey into three smaller components lessened the feelings of uncertainty I had. Our preacher shared:

- Faith is built; it is not just something we are given.

- Following Jesus is usually done one step of trust at a time.

- Small steps of faith allow the Lord to reveal Himself.

I also learned that everyone starts off with a learning curve regarding faith. Some people learn early in their life, while some of us wait until our mid-forties or later to truly recognize all that God has to offer.

SEEING TRUTH CLEARLY

What would happen if I truly got out of the way and allowed God to work in my life? I wanted to open my heart fully to Him, but still sometimes I struggled with fear, reminded of the pain I encountered when I had opened my heart to someone before.

I began praying for God's strength to help me do what He was asking me to do. If I slipped, if I sinned, I went to Him quickly in repentance and faith for Him to bring my heart back in line with His. I wanted to learn from Him and from my experiences.

As I gave the Lord the final say about when and how things happened in my world, and even what needed to be done, I found a new level of freedom. These steps of faith allowed the Lord to start revealing himself to me in the most unusual ways. Small wins became bigger wins. Bigger wins became more frequent.

LEARNING TO BE LED BY THE HOLY SPIRIT

Through the power of the Holy Spirit, who is spiritually active within God's children, God is always at work. I found that if I allowed Him to, He would help strengthen my thoughts, calm my fears and anxieties, and help me distinguish between right and wrong. If I allowed Him to, He would guide me, teach me, strengthen me when I'm weak, and lead in my interactions with other people.

The Holy Spirit provided me with the power to tackle the difficult parts of my recovery. When things got too tough and I wanted to give up, the Holy Spirit kept me fighting the voices of my abuser and the devil in my head.

During my uncertainty in figuring out my journey to domestic violence survivor, the Holy Spirit directed my path, allowing me to accomplish God's will within my doubting and uncertain perspective of my world. I find it amazing that God is so sincere about drawing me to Himself that He provided the Holy Spirit to enable, assist, and guide me.

When I first came back to my faith, I found it frustrating to know that other people could gauge their lives off the Bible, their prayers, and hearing God's voice. This is what I wanted! At first this task seemed too overwhelming, but in learning to trust God, learn His Word, and be quiet before Him, I was able to do this.

Looking back on my journey, I realize that when I surrendered my world to God through believing in Jesus Christ, the Holy Spirit was there, but it was as if He was squashed into a tiny place in my heart that was surrounded by the enormous strength of the residual effects of the abuse.

But that initially "small" Holy Spirit exercised His muscles to remove my abuser and all his darkness out of my heart and allowed me to grow in my faith. I could not move my abuser's lies on my own. I could not grow in my faith on my own. I needed the help of the Lord God working for me, in me, and through me.

FINAL THOUGHTS:
LIVING ON GOD'S TIMELINE

THE THOUGHT PROCESS OF LIVING ON GOD'S TIMELINE

Ecclesiastes 3:1-4: *"There is a time for everything, and a season for every activity under the heavens: a time to be born and a time to die, a time to plant and a time to uproot, a time to kill and a time to heal, a time to tear down and a time to build, a time to weep and a time to laugh, a time to mourn and a time to dance."*

I know there is no comparison between God and my abuser, yet my deep-rooted feelings of abandonment didn't just disappear when my abuser left the children and me. My feelings of desertion, my belief I was unworthy of love, these convictions were buried so deep in my subconscious that I needed to deliberately work on bringing them to the surface so I could tackle them. I discovered these buried emotions only when I purposefully focused on living according to God's timeline.

God's loving prodding enabled me to peel back the destroyed layers of my thought processes so I could see Satan's distortions for what they were and so I could begin rebuilding my process of reflection. Although it surely wasn't my goal when I started my journey to domestic violence survivor, I now see the central problem that needed to be corrected was retraining how I think.

How did I strengthen my ability to relinquish control of the events in my life and allow God's timeline to become the foundation for my decision-making? A few of my strategies include:

- Praying specifically for patience as I wait for God to reveal His timeline;

- Immediately switching my thought process if I begin planning for something that I'm not sure will occur.

- Deciding not to make decisions based on an internet search. It's easy for me to become distracted with reading something that then gets me self-diagnosing an ailment or figuring out how to answer something God has whispered to me. I have learned that for me, God prefers to use the Bible and humans as His messengers. I also found that sometimes decisions are made through indecision. Doing nothing can sometimes be a viable option, but it is also sometimes a way to demonstrate a lack of trust toward God's timeline. Just because I decide to allow God to guide me through my life's events doesn't mean I can sit back and wait for God to make everything happen. I am still required to move forward as He directs, but I do it knowing that while I am working on the task at hand, God is working within me.

I'm thankful for my church, doctor, specialists, and multiple therapists, the team that has supported, and in some cases, continues to support my transformation to domestic violence survivor. My experience leads me to believe we need to be educated on the multiple facets of our recovery effort so that the best plan of action can be put together to benefit us where we are in our journey. And, like all good plans of action, the strategies need to be adjusted as events change. Daily, my upkeep plan has included my medication, healthy diet, breathing and stretching, exercise, and my quiet times with the Lord. During so many lonely days, I knew I could trust God and confide my secret with Him. I found God always available and willing to talk, listen, and just be there with me.

THE STRENGTH OF LIVING ON GOD'S TIME LINE

As I've trusted in God, He has provided me with the strength to tackle my journey, fight the hard battles in my mind, and clean up after the devil's spiritual warfare.

Accepting Jesus into my life has provided me with an entirely new outlook on life. This new Spirit within me provides me the strength to look at every aspect of my thinking to retrain my thought process. Knowing that I follow God's guidance, even allowing for the twists and turns along the way, keeps my conscious clear against any attacks the devil might throw my way.

As I put on the armor of God described in Ephesians 6, I find that Jesus Christ Himself is the most powerful weapon against my lack of self-confidence, my lack of trust, my doubt, and my inability to figure out what to do.

The more I read and understand the Bible the more I am amazed at the power and strength of God's grace. His ability to completely transform hurt, wandering souls into people He uses to promote the growth of His kingdom is so amazing to me.

THE REWARD OF LIVING ON GOD'S TIMELINE

I see how God's timeline has led me to where I am today. I can also see how there were times when I thought I was ready to move forward, but God kept me in a holding pattern.

It is amazing to remember that when God moved me, then and only then could I say I was truly ready to take another step forward.

Learning how to live on God's timeline has come with lots of patience exercises for me, and I admit it continues to be difficult to do. But I love the thought of living in a world where I can enjoy life while waiting for the next piece to unfold. It's so much better than wasting so much time with unnecessary planning.

My challenge: plan only for those things that God has told me to plan for. This frees up a lot of my thoughts!

I realize that to devote my life 100 percent to God, I need to trust Him for what and when things are going to occur in my life.

There was no reason for me to do all the work to become a survivor unless all my negative, non-biblical thought processes were completely removed. Learning to live on God's timeline means handing over all power and influence, not only regarding what happens in my world, but also regarding how it happens.

It means that I trust Him as He guides me through life's events. I trust that the work I completed to break the cycle of violence is going to bring positive changes to the lineage of my children and their families. Regardless of what my kids' future holds, I know in my heart that I followed God's guidance and never gave up trying to beat the odds that were stacked against me.

What's the greatest reward I found living on God's timeline? The most valuable reward to me is the peace I've experienced. This calmness allows me to enjoy the life God provides for me as I wait for His next direction. The last residual piece of busyness in my mind is defeated and destroyed.

GOD CAN USE ANYBODY

If you doubt that God can use you to make dramatic changes in His world, remember that after Jesus died, rose again, and ascended back to heaven, He left his ministry to be carried on by His disciples—twelve ordinary men. These twelve men didn't have theological training and were not well known. There were common people, fishermen, a tax collector, one person from noble heritage, two brothers from a wealthy family. As far as we know, none of the twelve disciples had any training in the ways of God before Jesus called them to walk with Him.

The difference was that they had been with Jesus and on Pentecost they were filled with the Holy Spirit.

My low self-esteem, self-doubt, and anxiety-stricken personality make me a far more likely candidate for being a victim than a survivor. I was physically, emotionally, and sexually abused for so long that I honestly didn't know a different kind of world existed or was even available for me.

But God—not alcohol, a job, a relationship, money, or anything else—showed me the way to calmness and contentment in my life. Nothing else in the world saved me as God's love and grace did.

I have no special abilities or qualities that make me a better candidate for becoming a domestic violence survivor.

But I have been with Jesus, and He has given me His Holy Spirit.

I pray my journey aids in your own ability to transform from domestic violence victim to domestic violence survivor.

Blessings and prayers to all,
Sue

ABOUT THE AUTHOR

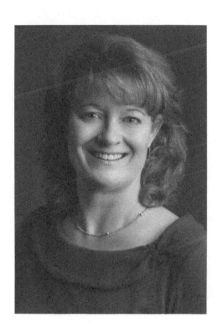

LTC (R) Sue Parisher served twenty-one honorable years on active duty, living a double life of capability and accomplishment in the service while enduring brutality and abusiveness in her twenty-year oppressive marriage. You can visit her blog at https://www.recoveringfrom-domesticviolence.com/

Rebecca Davis is a writer and editor with a passion to help the oppressed. She is the collaborating author for *Tear Down This Wall of Silence: Dealing with Sexual Abuse in Our Churches* (with Dale Ingraham) and *Unholy Charade: Unmasking the Domestic Abuser in the Church* (with Jeff Crippen). Among Rebecca's solo books is *Untwisting Scriptures that were used to tie you up, gag you, and tangle your mind.*